The Fat Girl
from Hollyoaks

Mikyla Dodd

The Fat Girl from Hollyoaks

HODDER &
STOUGHTON

First published in Great Britain in 2007 by Hodder & Stoughton
A division of Hodder Headline

1

A CIP catalogue record for this title is available from the British Library

ISBN 978 0 340 93547 7

Typeset in Sabon by Hewer Text UK Ltd, Edinburgh
Printed and bound by Mackays of Chatham Ltd, Chatham, Kent

Hodder Headline's policy is to use papers that are natural, renewable
and recyclable products and made from wood grown in sustainable
forests. The logging and manufacturing processes are expected to
conform to the environmental regulations of the country of origin.

Hodder & Stoughton Ltd
A division of Hodder Headline
338 Euston Road
London NW1 3BH

To Ella

Contents

PROLOGUE
The Moment in the Mirror

24 stone 7 pounds

Too tall, too fat, too ginger. That's what I've been for most of my life: at home, at school and especially in the one area I was passionate about – acting.

But not today. Today it was all going to change. Goodbye, boring office job; goodbye, Blackburn; goodbye, failure. The bright lights of London and the gleaming lens of a movie camera beckoned. Today London, tomorrow Hollywood.

It was October 1998 and I could barely contain myself. 'My career as a real live actress is about to begin,' I whispered. I walked through the smart South London council estate looking for the building where it was all going to happen. My heart pounded with a mixture of fear, nerves and excitement.

The estate was nothing like the rough places in my home town of Blackburn. It was full of smart townhouses and flats brightened up with window boxes and hanging baskets. Most estates in Blackburn were rough and scuffed with not a flower in sight. They were places where nobody ventured after dark unless they absolutely had to. I hadn't visited London very often and I was impressed that even the council estates were more upmarket than ours in the North. It all added to the glamour of my imminent movie stardom.

When I arrived at the address I'd written down, though, the setting wasn't quite what I'd envisaged for my big break. The venue was about as far from the Warner Brothers lot in Hollywood as it was possible to get, but I understood that in life things didn't always work out exactly as I hoped and dreamt they would. As I stood outside the rather dilapidated building, I told myself that this moment was the beginning of the rest of my life. I wasn't going to let anything or anyone spoil this for me, not even the giant sign above the door that said, 'Sumo Wrestling Centre of Excellence.' Yes, that's right. My first big role – literally – was going to be as a female sumo wrestler.

The film was called *Secret Society*. It was billed as a romantic comedy about a group of female factory workers who were all keen sumo wrestlers in their spare time. The film was about empowering overweight women and making them feel sensual and beautiful. When I heard about the concept, I was very excited. I thought it would be a chance for me and my supersized body not only to become socially acceptable for the first time ever, but to become famous too. After all, there was a huge amount of kudos attached to appearing in a film, especially for an unknown like me.

At the time I was a size 28 and rarely felt sensual or beautiful, with tyres of fat lolling between the top of my Bridget Jones knickers and my polyester 46DD over-the-shoulder-boulder-holder. I had originally been offered the lead role, but because it involved a peculiar kind of nudity – allowing cat's whiskers to be drawn on to my naked breasts

– I declined it and instead accepted a lesser role as a member of the sumo sisterhood, which meant that my overgrown puppies stayed firmly inside my bra. I was going to get paid £12,000 for four months' work – more money than I'd ever earned in my life, and for doing something I loved. I couldn't believe my luck. I probably would have been paid twice that if I'd allowed my pale-pink nipples to double up as kittens' noses, but even if I'd been offered serious money, that was never going to happen.

The Sumo Wrestling Centre of Excellence looked like a disused garage with wooden decking outside. Was I expected to knock on the door, or simply walk in?

I stepped straight inside and saw an older man in a tracksuit walking across the hall. He looked strong and wiry and didn't have an ounce of spare flesh on his lithe frame. I'd been told to ask for a man called Sid who would be training me and the other wannabe sumo wrestlers before filming began. I assumed this was the man who had agreed to take on me and nine other giant mamas and turn us into mean, if not lean, fighting machines.

'Oh, hello, are you Sid?' I said, trying to sound bright and confident.

'Yes, I am, and you're . . . ?'

'Mikyla, Mikyla Dodd,' I said, extending my hand. He shook it vigorously.

'Well, it's very nice to meet you, Mikyla. Come this way. The others haven't arrived yet.'

Sid appeared entirely at ease with my size. Usually when people met me for the first time, particularly if they hadn't had any prior warning that I was a 'big girl', they were unable to stop themselves looking me up and down and from side to side. But Sid didn't gawp at all; he just grinned and gestured for me to follow him.

I had always thought that anything to do with films would be full of bustle and people, but this place was eerily deserted. The large training room had chilly concrete floors and the laboured, sweaty smell of a school gym. At one end of the room was a complete wall of mirrors. From the far end of the room, I thought my reflection looked pretty good, and I admired my curves. But as I walked closer to the mirror, I seemed to grow larger and larger, until eventually I became as big as a house – a three-bedroom semi, to be precise. I shuddered and hurriedly turned my back on the unforgiving mirrors. I managed to erase the super-fat image of myself from my mind – something I'd become an expert at during all the years of being in denial about my size.

I focused my thoughts on the training ahead. If I was being taught something that interested me, I was a quick and dedicated student. I vowed that learning to sumo-wrestle was something I would apply myself to 100 per cent. I liked the look of Sid. The twinkle in his eye suggested that he had a good sense of humour. I decided that he would be a demanding teacher but also a fair one. As with most people I liked, I wanted to win his approval.

Gradually the other women filed in. We had all been asked to wear loose, comfortable clothing to train in, but the baggy tracksuit bottoms and T-shirts didn't conceal very much as far as the weight of my fellow actresses was concerned. I had always assessed other women's bodies – particularly large women. Were they fatter than me? More or less in proportion? Why were they fat? Did they overeat, or was their weight down to a medical condition? Did I look better or worse when stood next to them? As they walked around the room, I began my usual fat mental arithmetic, noticing instantly that these women were all bigger than me. One woman had a skinny face and shoulders, but from nowhere a huge belly mushroomed into view. I gave myself a bonus point when I compared myself with her – at least my body was in proportion.

I felt worried for some of the women – they were so large that their weight must have been a strain on their health. Did they take up an entire double bed all by themselves? I wondered. I struggled to get into a theatre or a plane seat, but I thought that they probably wouldn't even be allowed on to a plane. Usually my justifying sums went something like this: 'Maybe I've got more muscle than they have and that's why I look big. Well, I'm a lot taller than they are, so I can afford to carry more weight. I'm quite pretty, and having a pretty face makes up for a couple of stone. I've always been able to make people laugh, and maybe that makes up for being fat.'

After an overview from Sid about the importance of inner as well as outer strength, Sid asked us to line up facing the mirror so that we could practise a basic move – the classic stamping of feet and shaking of thighs. Looking at our reflection, we made quite a sight. All ten of us had differently distributed undulating piles of flesh vibrating under our T-shirts and tracksuit bottoms. Upper arms shook with ripples of excess flesh, thighs trembled, and bellies and buttocks looked tight and swollen, as if someone had crept around with a balloon pump and secretly inflated us with so much air that we were all at risk of popping.

Only it wasn't air; it was pure fat. As I looked back and forth at the other women's reflections and my own, cold horror crept over me.

I had been a chubby child, and when I entered my teens, my plumpness increased so that I was officially fat. I had continued putting on weight for the next few years and had never deluded myself that I wasn't fat; I accepted that I was fat. Sometimes I was perfectly happy being fat, and at other times I felt absolutely wretched. But for the first time the juxtaposition of my reflection with these women who were morbidly obese made me see that there was no difference between them and me. I was appalled and disgusted with myself in a way I never had been before. I knew that there was big and then there was 'Oh, my bloody God, what is that?' and somehow, without me noticing, I had travelled from the former group to the latter. I wanted to burst into tears on the spot, but as often happens to me in a crisis, I went on to automatic pilot. 'Put your tears away and deal with this later,' I said to myself sternly.

When I went home that night, I sobbed and sobbed at the body I had been dragging around and managing to ignore but now knew was gross, thanks to that revelatory moment in the mirror.

I had often idly thought about losing weight. I had tried every diet under the sun – briefly – and had always gone back to my old ways. But there was a sudden difference inside me after I lined up alongside the sumo women, a kind of electric shock to the soul. I knew that it would be impossible to diet while I was working on a film, because in order to diet I needed to be in a daily routine in which I could buy and cook my own food and eat at regular times.

That was never going to happen on a film set with the catering crew serving up stodgy meals. Also, continuity was a major issue when filming – I couldn't afford to be seen to shrink from one frame to the next.

I vowed that the day the final frame of the film was shot, for the first time in my life I was going to seriously lose weight. I promised myself that I wasn't going to give up until I was back to looking like the real person that was trapped in this mountainous body. I longed to be a comfortable size 16. I wanted to shed weight not for my acting career, or to attract a man, but for myself. I knew that I deserved better than abusing my body day after day by gorging on supersize fast-food meals and stacks of cakes and biscuits. I knew that it was time to start respecting myself, and with a post-film regime of exercise, lean protein and piles of vegetables, that was exactly what I was going to do.

I

'As Long as He's Not Ginger . . .'

7 pounds 12 ounces

I was a baby who was desperately wanted by my mum but not so much by my dad. My mum had always adored babies, while my dad wasn't at all interested in experiencing parenthood.

My mum had had a strange childhood. Her own mother had married the love of her life, but tragically he died of meningitis when my mum, Valerie, was two and a half. My nan, a Scouser, and my mum were evacuated towards the end of the war. The local butcher wooed her by giving her the best cuts of meat and asked her to marry him. My nan didn't love him, but urged on by her mother and sisters, who told her, 'You won't do better,' and reluctant to struggle on as a single mother, she agreed. After the marriage my nan gave birth to a son.

The butcher was unnecessarily cruel to my mum, his newly acquired stepdaughter. At sixteen he placed her under curfew, and if she didn't come home on time, he locked her out or, even worse, defaced or destroyed one of her treasured possessions. She got a job on the perfume counter at Boots when rationing was still in place and perfume was a relatively rare and precious commodity. One night when she came home later than she was supposed to, he poured her perfume down the sink to punish her. Not surprisingly my mum was keen to leave her oppressive home. To get away and broaden her horizons, when she was eighteen she decided to go to Guernsey with some girlfriends for the summer. It was there that she met Archie, an older man, fifteen years older to be precise, who swept her off her feet. Prone to the odd bout of impulsive behaviour, she rang my nan to announce that she wouldn't be coming home and to request her belongings be sent on to her.

Mum married Archie and had three children in quick succession: two daughters – Ella in October 1960, then Sam in September 1962 – and a son, Jay, in the summer of 1964. Archie, who had at first seemed so alluring and such a great alternative to life at home with her stepdad, became distant towards her. He began to lose his appeal once he started to slump by the fireside with his pipe and slippers. I often wonder whether an older man would make a good partner for me – somebody wiser who could give me advice and who would be more accepting of my curvaceous figure than a younger man – but whenever I say this to my mum she's always quick to point out the downside of such couplings.

She decided she wanted to divorce Archie, but didn't realise that because she was not a Guernsey resident born and bred, she had no automatic right of custody to the children. With a heavy heart she returned to live with my nan, visiting the children regularly. After eighteen months Archie agreed with her that he wasn't doing a particularly good job juggling parenthood with work and allowed her to take the children back to England.

Several years later, my mum met my dad, Glenn, at a house party somewhere on the Wirrel. At the time he was still married to his childhood sweetheart, Yvonne, known as Vonnie. He and Vonnie were running a pub together in Cheshire, and although their relationship had broken down, the two of them remained good pals. When my mum met my dad, in 1975, Ella was fifteen, Sam thirteen, and Jay eleven. They were by this point settled in Darwen, near Blackburn, and my dad was living in his home town of Nantwich, Cheshire. Their relationship involved a lot of commuting between the two places. After six months of long-distance passion, my mum said, 'Glenn, I'd love to have a baby.' She was thirty-six and very keen to fit one more in before she got too old. She never applied any pressure on my dad to commit himself to her, but hoped he would rise to the challenge of parenthood.

My dad was horrified. Fathering a child didn't feature in his life plan. He has never particularly liked children – babies yes, but children, no – and didn't hesitate to tell my mum this. My mum was sure that she could win him round, though, so she coaxed and cajoled, using every tool of persuasion available. She knew that my dad disliked children but wasn't going to let that little detail stand in her way. She wanted a baby and by hook or by crook she was going to get one. She loved my dad and it made perfect sense to her to have her baby with the man she loved.

'No way, Val. Forget it. You've already got three children. Why do you want any more? We're fine as we are.'

'Look, Glenn, I've brought up three children single-handed, and if needs be I'll bring up another one on my own. You don't have to do anything if you don't want to. I'll be forty in a few years – I'm running out of time.'

And so they argued back and forth, back and forth. Eventually my mum got her way and got pregnant. But she had a miscarriage.

My dad said, 'Maybe it's a sign that you and I aren't meant to have a baby.'

'No it's not,' said my mum firmly, and within a few months was pregnant with me.

My mum was absolutely convinced that once I arrived in the world my dad's heart would melt and he would be transformed into a doting parent. During the pregnancy he seemed to come round at least partially to the idea.

'It might not be too bad if it's a boy, as long as he's not ginger,' said my dad hesitantly. He had been a ginger-haired child and was teased mercilessly for it, and he was keen to have a boy so that his family name could continue.

By the time I emerged from the womb, on 29 September 1977, I'd already committed two big blunders – I was a girl, and I had a fine dusting of ginger on my scalp.

In the early months of my life my dad appeared to have overcome this double disappointment. According to my mum, he was good with me. He bounced me up and down on his fat stomach, endlessly singing 'The Grand Old Duke of York' to me.

When I look back at pictures of myself as a baby, I think, God, I was an ugly bugger! I had a very big head with the same deep, bumpy forehead as my dad, and to make matters worse my head wasn't in proportion with my body. My skin was so pale it was almost transparent, and the whole Mikyla package was crowned with a mop of carrot-coloured hair. For the time being, however, I was a welcome baby.

When I was born, Ella was seventeen, Sam was fifteen and Jay was thirteen. As a baby, Ella adored me. She was almost old enough to be my mother. She put me in a pram and used to walk up and down the street with me, telling everyone who peeped into the pram to coo at me that I was her baby. She treated me like a little doll, dressing me in four or five different outfits a day and changing my nappy. She wasn't a jealous person and didn't resent my arrival in any way.

Once I began exerting my personality, all the abstract dislike my dad had had for me pre-conception and during the pregnancy returned in full force. My mum's optimistic belief that my dad would adore me just as much as she did was sadly misplaced. He knew his own mind. His outlook is very black and white, with no room for shades of grey, and he doesn't have much patience. By the time I was six months old I was a thorn in his side, a constant irritation that prevented him from doing lots of things he had become accustomed to doing in his previous child-free existence. He regularly shook his head or rolled his eyes, exasperated by the level of attention I demanded. Sometimes he got so fed up with me that he told me to 'just shut up and go away'.

I'm very much my father's daughter and I know how much I hate being coerced into doing something. For him, having me was a bit like being dragged around Alton Towers at its busiest with no end in sight. My dad loved dining out in nice restaurants, spur-of-the-moment holidays and getting peace and quiet whenever he wanted it. I got in the way of all that.

In the face of opposition to my existence from my dad, my mum showered me with more than enough love for both of them. When she had been a single parent bringing up my three older half-siblings, who were close together in age, it had been challenging enough just getting through the day and she had rarely had the energy or resources to devote quality time to them. By the time she had me, however, her circumstances were very different. Her older three children were partly self-sufficient and she had a lot of 'mother energy' to devote to me. I know that I got the very best out of her.

She showed an incredible softness towards me and was very affectionate, always hugging and cuddling me. She was less objective about me than about the other three, particularly when it came to defending my misdemeanours from my dad's sharp tongue. From a very early age I was aware of the dissatisfaction my dad felt with my existence, and I was equally aware of my mum's adoration of me. It was a strange, unbalanced feeling, like walking through puddles with one foot protected by a sturdy wellington boot, the other covered only in a thin sock.

My mum felt guilty about my dad's attitude because he had given her due warning of his views about having a child before I was even conceived. When I had annoyed him, however many times she tried to intervene on my behalf, he would retort, 'Look, Valerie, I didn't want to be a parent, and I never said I'd be a good one.'

She was deeply saddened that he didn't share her joy

over me. It was unfortunate that of all the people in the world who could have been my dad's kid he had to get me. Not only was I female and ginger, I was spirited and demanding. It appeared I was everything he didn't want and more.

2
This Is What Happens When You're Bored

3 stone 2 pounds

I can't remember a time when I didn't think about food. It penetrated every level of my consciousness from a very early age. As soon as I had learnt to talk in reasonably full and coherent sentences, I demanded to know from my mum when the next meal was and what it consisted of so that I could a) look forward to it, b) know how long I had to wait for it, and c) offer my objections in advance if it wasn't something I fancied and then try to secure a more delicious substitute.

My love of food and mischief sometimes combined with disastrous consequences. When I was about eighteen months old, I was in the kitchen and my beady eyes fastened on a large and gooey chocolate cake that Ella, Sam and Jay had bought for our mum as a Mother's Day treat. It was a sponge cake crowned with thick, dark frosting and the words 'We love you, Mum' in spidery white icing. As the icing glistened in the light, the temptation became too great for me. I dug my hands deep into the cake almost up to my elbows and began scooping handfuls of the heavenly dark, sweet stuff into my mouth.

My sister Sam had gone to the toilet during my attack on

the cake. By the time she emerged from the bathroom and caught me red-handed, most of my upper body and every millimetre of my face had turned chocolate brown. She looked aghast at my act of unintentional sabotage. She ran down to the baker's, bought another, smaller cake and crammed it into the chasm that I'd opened up in the middle of the first cake. The tale became famous in our family and was retold many times. 'I wouldn't mind but I'd only nipped in for a number one,' was Sam's comment.

Because my mum worked full-time running a florists, I spent a lot of time in her shop. A lot of the time, apart from Christmas and Valentine's Day, the shop was quiet and entertainment was scarce. I made beds for myself out of the flower boxes and used the satin backcloth meant for funeral flowers to dress up in. As soon as I was old enough to hold a pair of scissors responsibly, Mum taught me how to trim flower stems: 'Always cut them on the slant, Mik, and then if they're thirsty they'll be able to have a nice long drink.'

In my early days at the flower shop, my mum was potty-training me, and on one occasion she almost died of embarrassment when a sales rep came to the shop. From the moment I could string a couple of words together, I loved saying things to the customers and the reps. So I toddled up to the sales rep in my chintzy dress and said, beaming, 'Hiya, hiya.'

The rep smiled at me and then carried on talking to my mum. She was selling these pastel-coloured plastic bowls intended to hold flowers and was telling my mum how they were the best thing since sliced bread when it came to the art of arranging flowers. When she put her lovely plastic bowls down on the floor, however, I assumed they were potties, lifted up my dress and promptly peed into one of them. Well, it certainly looked like a potty to me! My mum was mortified but managed to keep her cool. She looked first at me and then at the sales rep and said, 'I'll take that one, please. What other colours do they come in?'

My mum and dad took me on holiday to Italy when I was a toddler and I became very popular with the waitresses. I sat in my high chair, and every day when they said to me, '*Zuppa* or pasta?' I would squeal, 'Pasta!' with delight. Even then, starchy carbs were a favourite. They found it hilarious and endearing that such a young child could order from the menu, and each evening after I'd finished eating they swept me out of my high chair and danced around the restaurant with me singing, '*Bella bambina.*'

The house where my love of food really developed was an old grey stone house in Billinge Avenue, Blackburn. It wasn't the first house I lived in as a child, but it's the one I remember best. I liked being in the centre of the house in Billinge Avenue – in the kitchen, where my mum cooked solid, wholesome meals, or the TV room, or my mum's quiet sitting room, which was a TV-free zone. I don't like to miss out on any kind of action now and I didn't like to then either. From the moment I became aware of the things going on around me I wanted to experience them first hand.

I avoided the top and bottom of the house. At the bottom, down a chilly flight of stone steps, was the cellar. My dad was a builder who specialised in damp-proofing and he stored barrels of the damp-proofing chemical Re-mtox in the dank, dark cellar. I refused to go down there without a grown-up. My mum used the cellar as a workshop to cut stems off the flowers she had risen at 3 a.m. to drive to Manchester to collect. I wasn't aware as a child just how hard my mum worked. She was usually in the cellar before I woke up, so I rarely saw it brightened up by her cheerful, busy presence.

Even the garden at the house in Billinge Avenue was gloomy. There was a huge weeping willow that overshadowed everything else, and a rickety, rusty swing, which looked as if it had been there for generations. Playing there by myself made me feel miserable. I had a pair of red and silver roller skates, which I was very proud of. The ground was uneven and sloped, so I tumbled over in them so many times that my hips and ample bum turned black and blue, but I was determined to keep trying. In the end my dad tied a cushion to my bottom with string to soften my fall. And after what I considered to be a superhuman level of perseverance, I mastered the tricky art of roller skating on a hill.

As well as the garden and the cellar, the other place I didn't like going to was my playroom in the attic. On the face of it, it was kind of my dad to build it for me, but I got very lonely up there. I wanted to be with the rest of the family, but often my dad would try to banish me to there. The room used to be my brother Jay's bedroom, and when he moved out to go into the army at the age of sixteen, my dad converted it into the playroom. I was only three when Jay moved out and have no memories of him living in the house.

Jay was away in the army, Sam spent a lot of her time in Guernsey, where she knew people from her childhood, and so Ella was the only sibling I saw consistently. When I was little she lived at home, but even when she moved into her own place nearby I still saw her most days. As a result of the large age gap between me and my siblings and their partial or total absence from my daily life, I was often lonely at home. I vowed from a young age that if and when I had children I would have two close together so that they could keep each other company. To date I haven't had any children, but I still feel that very strongly.

'Why don't you go off and play now, Miky Dripping – that's why I built you a playroom, so you'd have some-where to play,' said my dad far too often. Whenever I dragged myself up the stairs to the attic, I sat and calculated what was the shortest possible time I could get away with spending up there. After half an hour or so I'd reappear with a hopeful expression on my face.

It was just before I started school, aged four, that I demonstrated an enthusiasm for performing. When my mum was in the bathroom putting on her make-up, I'd put down the lid of the toilet seat, climb up on to it and deliver my Oscar acceptance speech. I had seen the Oscars on TV and was very taken by the whole thing. I made what my mum tells me was a reasonable stab at an American accent. 'I'd like to thank everyone so much for this award,' I gushed. 'Especially my mom, who lives in London, England.'

'But I don't live in London,' my mum giggled.

'I know, but that's what Americans always say,' I replied.

I remember from this time that although my dad was frequently hostile towards me, he also showed me moments of great love and thoughtfulness. Because my dad was still married to Vonnie when I was born, even though their relationship was long over, he didn't tell his parents about me until I was three. Once they found out and came to terms with the fact that they had a surprise grandchild, he took me to visit them every week.

On Tuesdays I sat proudly next to my dad while he sang songs like 'Nobody's Child' and 'The Little Boy That Santa Claus Forgot'. Even though the songs weren't very cheerful, I loved hearing them because my dad was singing them especially for me. Sometimes I made requests. 'Please, Dad, will you sing the one about the train driver who crashes his train and dies?'

At that time Ella had moved back in with us, and I shared a room with her and her son, Rosco, who was three and a half years younger than me. Ella had met Rosco's father, Tony, in Guernsey. Like Sam, she still spent some of her time there. Tony was a sailor. I think Ella did love him but knew the relationship was doomed. They didn't live together before or after Rosco was born, and their relationship was very much an on-off affair.

I had always adored Ella, but I didn't feel any envy when Rosco arrived and she became absorbed with him. In fact the night Rosco was born was very exciting for me because I was allowed to stay up late and was bought some succulent, fatty takeaway fried chicken for the first time in my life. It was instant love on my part.

I loved helping Ella with Rosco, obediently fetching nappies and, more importantly, rusks. My reward for being so helpful was getting to eat one of the rusks. I must have been the oldest child in Blackburn eating rusks, and I learnt how to swallow them quickly before they got too soggy. In the early years I was very kind and gentle towards Rosco. I was a lonely child and I was overjoyed to have a playmate. Later on, though, things were less harmonious between us and we fought and squabbled. While I didn't mind Rosco being part of our family, I did resent it when my mum spent time with him because I wanted her all to myself.

I always got along well with Ella. She was the peace-keeper of the family, and I loved spending time with her even if we sat in companionable silence. She introduced me to the music she loved – singers like Luther Vandross and George Benson – and sometimes we danced around like idiots to it. Her health had always been fragile – she suffered from asthma and had had her large intestine removed due to ulcerative colitis. But on a day-to-day level her health was fine and she lived a normal life.

From the age of two I had been taller than other children my age. By the time I started school, aged four, I looked like the average seven-year-old. Looking so much older than I was, was a curse. Because I looked so mature, the family assumed I was more self-sufficient than I actually was, and complete strangers expected much more of me than a child of my age was capable of delivering. All I wanted was to be at the hub of family life, to have attention lavished on me and not to have to go it alone quite so often.

By this point, assumptions about my size were already firmly in place. I wasn't fat, but I was taller and broader than my classmates. Although I knew I was bigger than the other children, I didn't really mind and I didn't equate my size with how much I ate.

The head teacher at my primary school, aka Grotbags, took me aside on my first day and said in a way I think she hoped would comfort me that she had the perfect friend for me: 'Mikyla, I'd like you to meet Catherine. She's a big girl just like you and I'm sure the two of you will get on famously.'

Catherine had short, dark hair. She lived on a farm and smelt faintly of earth and manure. The two of us grew at the same rate and were nicknamed the Amazons. As luck would have it, we got along famously and I became fond of her farmy scent. She came from a family of four girls who all had to help out on the farm. I was glad that I didn't have to do any chores at home or have any responsibilities in the household, so I could devote all my energies to being a pain in the neck. I often got blamed for things at school because I was bigger than the other children and so stood out more, catching the teachers' eyes when they were trying to find a culprit – a curse that followed me around during my entire school career. Sometimes they blamed me correctly, but at other times I was accused of committing misdemeanours that had absolutely nothing to do with me.

Soon after I started school, my dad bought me a beautiful doll's house filled with miniature furniture. He also made a member of staff at Argos open scores of Cabbage Patch Doll boxes until he found one with red hair to match mine. As a child, it wasn't possible for me to fathom the complexity of my dad's attitude towards me. Children need consistency, and I couldn't understand how sometimes he showed me so much love and sometimes he seemed so cold towards me.

Two of the words my dad most hated to hear were 'I'm bored', so I tried to wait until he was out of the way before I uttered them. My dad had supersonic hearing and one day he heard me muttering about being bored from the next room. He blasted out of his chair and said, 'Right, that's it.' Enraged, he hurried up the stairs to my playroom.

My mum shot out from the kitchen when she heard the commotion.

'Glenn, what on earth are you doing?' she called.

My dad was standing angrily at the top of the stairs with my beloved doll's house in his arms. 'Bored, she says. We'll see how bored she gets when I give all her toys away to an orphanage.' He bundled the doll's house and some of my other toys into the back of his van and sped off. I was heartbroken and couldn't stop sobbing.

My mum wasn't sure if he was just trying to teach me a lesson and would be back at any moment with the toys still in the back of his van or if he was really serious about giving them away. It turned out to be the latter! He came home with the van empty and looking rather pleased with himself.

My mum spent several hours trying to wheedle out of him the location of the place where he had dumped my toys. She had a harder job on her hands than an MI5 official interrogating an enemy spy. But in the end my dad confessed, 'Stop nagging me, for God's sake – I took the stuff to the charity shop in the high street.'

That was all my mum needed to know. She grabbed my hand and we raced out to her car. By the time we arrived there the staff at the shop had displayed my doll's house in pride of place in the centre of the window. Horrified, I burst into floods of tears.

'Don't worry,' soothed my mum. 'Once we explain that it was all a horrible misunderstanding, I'm sure we'll get the doll's house back straight away.'

Well, she couldn't have been more wrong.

'I'm sorry, Mrs Dodd, we've already sold several items, and the rest of the stuff is now the property of the charity shop. If you want it back, you'll have to buy it.' I started sobbing again. My mum's mouth dropped open but she realised she had no alternative but to pay to get back what was left of my own toy collection.

I went home traumatised, clutching as many toys as I could fit into my arms. And I never did say I was bored again.

3
'New Clothes, New Mood'

5 stone 2 pounds

One of my clearest memories is of the Christmas that I was five. Jay was on leave from the army and had returned home in the early hours from a Christmas Eve party. This woke me up and I bounded out of bed overjoyed that Christmas Day had finally arrived, ripped open my presents and tried on the new clothes Santa had so cleverly chosen. Once the novelty wore off I ventured into Jay's room and cried out, 'Merry Christmas.' He noisily returned the greeting.

At this point my dad woke up and stormed into Jay's room, fuming and bleary-eyed. 'Stop that bloody racket now and get those new clothes off,' he said to me. 'I don't want to hear from you for at least another four hours.'

I retreated miserably to my bedroom and sat waiting patiently for four hours to pass. I was far too hyped up about Christmas to go back to sleep, but for the first time I did wonder whether Santa Claus actually existed.

The house in Billinge Avenue was set back from the busy main road, and always seemed to be cold. It was on a bend, which meant that Tom, the little boy next door, and I could stare at each other through our bedroom windows. My dad caught us once pressed against our respective windows, me lifting my nightie up to my chin, him with his pyjama trousers pulled down, playing 'I'll show you mine if you show me yours'.

I was still only five years old at the time, and I didn't even know that I'd done anything wrong, but my dad behaved as if he'd caught the two of us doing something horrific. He pulled me away from the window and yelled, 'Don't you dare go around revealing yourself like that. If I ever catch you doing something like that again, you'll really be in for it, young lady.'

My dad continued to run the pub he ran in Cheshire before he met my mum. That meant that he was away for part of the week and my mum was in charge at home. I felt much more at ease inviting friends back to play when he wasn't there.

Sometimes when my dad upset me I would throw a tantrum, then march up to my bedroom and pack my pyjamas and beloved punk-rocker doll into a little suitcase and announce that I was leaving. I never had the guts to carry out my threat, though, except once when I walked around the block three times but couldn't go any further as I wasn't allowed to cross the main roads! Usually I would emerge some time later hoping that nobody remembered the grand announcement about my imminent departure. Other times I would change my clothes while I was up in my bedroom in the mistaken belief that I would come across as a brand-new child. Sometimes this rigmarole was repeated four or five times a day, to the great annoyance of my mum, who had to pick up several discarded outfits from the floor. I favoured a Norma Desmond-style entrance, announcing, 'New clothes, new mood.'

Although I had been an ugly baby, I turned into a beautiful child with thick, red curly hair, big green eyes and cheeky dimples. I learnt how to make adults laugh, which was vital because I wanted everybody to love me. I also spent a lot more time around grown-ups than most children and learnt how to tune into adult conversations. I happily chatted to anyone I met. How I wasn't kidnapped, I'll never know.

I once asked my dad, 'What would you do if someone I started chatting to kidnapped me?'

'They'd have to pay us a ransom to take you back,' he said.

Everybody laughed. I tried to laugh too, but I felt wounded because young as I was, I understood that the joke was at my expense.

There was only one child who my dad seemed to soften towards. He was my cousin Kim's son, Alex. Alex was fascinated by my dad's van and his job as a builder. My dad found this very amusing and used to take Alex for rides in his van. Alex saw my dad as one of his heroes and he got excited at the mere mention of his name. I wondered if I would have fared better with my dad if I'd come into the world as a Michael rather than as a Mikyla. I'll never know.

One of the problems between my dad and me was that both of us wanted my mum all to ourselves. Because there was only one of her and two of us, things were never going to work out. Food was one way that I competed with my dad for my mum's affections. My mum didn't fill our house with junk food – she cooked wholesome, solid meals of the meat, potatoes and two vegetables variety.

When my mum put less food on my plate than on my dad's, I had a special look that I gave her. First I'd peer over to my dad's plate, then I'd look back to my plate. Next I put my chin on my chest and looked up at her with sad puppy-dog eyes. She usually put an extra spoonful or two on to my plate.

My mum never tried to restrict my eating when I was little. In response to my demands, she was giving me virtually adult portions, but she never thought my weight was an issue. My mum's own attitude to food seemed to be a pretty sensible one. She sat down and ate a reasonable-sized meal with the rest of us but never seemed to gorge herself. If she did put on a few pounds, she cut back, and although she wasn't slim as a sylph, she never became really overweight.

'She's training to be an Olympic eater,' my dad used to say about me, frequently and woundingly. His remarks failed to slim me down, though – quite the opposite. I ate more and more and I was already developing an addiction to the feeling I got when I had a full stomach.

Like my mum, my nan was another woman who adored me and fed me too much – and I'm not just talking about a couple of extra potatoes. Sometimes I went round to her flat after school. She was a shrunken woman with short grey hair, which she had set once a week. She often wore a paisley skirt and thick tights, and had a soft Scouse accent. She lived on the eleventh floor of a tall block of flats, and as soon as she heard me pressing the buzzer, she sprang into action chopping potatoes and heating oil in a pan to cook chips for me. My nan's chips always tasted so good – hot, fat and crispy with oil.

When I got back home, my mum always asked me, 'Have you eaten at your nan's?' Without hesitation I'd reply, 'Not much,' in the hope that I'd get another meal. As well as being keen to eat more food, I hated the thought of missing out on some action while the others sat round the table.

Although there wasn't an endless supply of sweets, crisps and chocolates at home, my nan used to visit every weekend and without fail would give me a goodie bag containing a Taxi bar, a Trio, a Blue Riband and various packets of crisps as well as Horlicks tablets, which I adored. Needless to say, I always demolished whatever she brought for me.

As my appetite increased, my sister Sam moved in the opposite direction. She was so completely obsessed with her body weight that she didn't pay much attention to mine. We didn't know much about eating disorders when Sam developed hers and certainly hadn't ever heard the word 'anorexia'. Her troubles had begun at the age of eighteen, when she had fallen in love with a footballer who played for Blackburn Rovers. This was in the days before Jack Walker and before footballers started to get paid millions, but locally Blackburn Rovers were big news.

Sam has always been very beautiful and was lots of fun, so it wasn't hard for this footballer to fall in love with her. But his father was totally opposed to the relationship, anxious that it would divert his talented son from his football career. He strongly advised him to end the relationship, which he eventually did. Sam is a sensitive soul at the best of times and she was absolutely devastated by this. She couldn't cure her broken heart, and her misery was compounded by the fact that the way the relationship ended was so entirely beyond her control. In a bid to exert control over at least one area of her life, she began to starve herself, restricting herself to cold, dry pitta bread. She locked herself in her room, endlessly playing Karen Carpenter songs – she idolised her. My mum left the pitta bread on a plate outside Sam's room and hoped for the best. She thought the whole thing was part of a heartbroken phase that Sam was going through and played it down in the belief that that way it would pass more quickly.

Sam learnt from articles written about Karen Carpenter that taking laxatives was one way of keeping her weight low and decided to copy her. We had no idea she was doing this, and on the occasions when she did appear to eat normally we were all relieved. If we'd known that she was rushing off to the loo to purge herself whenever she did eat a normal meal, we would have been far more worried. While Sam's weight dropped dangerously low several times, causing her to be hospitalised, it was clear during this period that her mind was severely unbalanced. She managed to conceal her lack of eating quite well from us by cooking all of us delicious meals but then hardly eating anything herself. To this day Sam still has an unusual relationship with food, and years of laxative abuse have certainly taken a toll on her health.

My dad loved going out to restaurants with my mum, but she often insisted on taking me along too. They took me on holiday to Italy for the second time when I was five. My mum and dad left me in the hotel room while they went down for dinner. I hated being left out and felt very bored stuck in the hotel room. One morning when we went down for breakfast in the hotel I was feeling particularly disgruntled about having been left by myself the night before and decided I was going to annoy my mum and dad by eating and eating and eating until I was fit to burst. I gorged myself on cereal, hunks of olive-oil bread and slices of cold meat, all washed down with strawberry yoghurt. Even my mum, who usually indulged my large appetite, noticed. My dad, in his usual hard manner, said, 'Don't you think you've had enough there, Mik?' I defiantly carried on chewing and scooped up my next mouthful.

After breakfast my mum and dad, their friends Johnny and Denise and me jumped into the car and began a journey along some very windy roads to reach the next town we had planned to visit. My stomach was alarmingly full – to the point of bursting.

'My tummy hurts,' I said quietly to my mum, hoping my dad wouldn't hear.

'Shh,' soothed Mum. 'Just look straight ahead and you'll probably feel better.'

Her advice didn't work. Suddenly I was very, very sick – not any old puking, but a magnificent fountain of projectile-vomiting, which splattered all over my dad. Unpleasant as it was being so sick, I did later that day smile to myself, remembering my dad climbing out of the car and hopelessly trying to sponge himself clean.

There was some kind of justice for him a couple of days later when we stopped at a small inn to eat. The waitress spoke no English. My mum and dad ordered the same meal and then my dad asked for '*poco*' for me, thinking that meant 'small'. However, when the food arrived, there was a meal for my mum, a meal for my dad but nothing for me.

My mum and dad decided that the waitress had interpreted 'poco' to be 'porco' and my dad's request as 'Nothing for the little pig'!

Jay, my brother, could sometimes be almost as hurtful to me as my dad. He never did much to make me feel that I was part of the family, and at one point he referred to me as his 'stepsister', which alienated me further. I wanted to cry out, 'I'm not your stepsister. If you want to be technically correct about it, I'm your half-sister, but really I'm just your bloody sister.'

I never said that at the time, but did blurt it out when drunk one night. These days Jay and I are very close, but when I was a child we really didn't get along at all. The two men I desperately wanted to impress when I was a little girl were my dad and my brother, and neither of them made it easy.

As a family, despite my difficulties with my dad and Jay, we did have fun. One family friend was a pleasant but increasingly forgetful old lady called Mrs Tattershall. It became a tradition to invite her round to our house for Christmas lunch. When she wasn't looking, we all laughed at her eccentric presents – a box of half-eaten chocolates that she'd rummaged in her attic for, or socks that moths had nibbled holes in, or a half-drunk bottle of Baileys. Ella would start laughing and her infectious giggle had a domino effect on the rest of us. My mum frantically tried to hush us in case Mrs Tattershall realised we were laughing at her, but thankfully she never did.

She also seemed immune to the rough and tumble of dining *chez* Dodd. Several strands of conversation would coexist chaotically across the table, and anyone whose contribution was deemed not particularly interesting would be knocked down smartly. If someone was in the middle of a boring, long-winded tale, one of us would say scathingly, 'Will this take long?'

Mrs Tattersall simply nodded as the banter boomeranged relentlessly back and forth. Joining in was quite simply not an option for her and she smiled blankly as jokes and caustic comments whirred around her.

Meanwhile life had changes in store for Ella and Sam. Ella's relationship with Tony, Rosco's father, had been very much off for a while, but then he begged her to take him back and marry him in Guernsey. She agreed but regretted it even before she walked down the aisle. It was a double wedding, with my sister Sam the other bride – the first one that had ever taken place in Guernsey. Sam had also met the man she'd agreed to marry in Guernsey. Ella was twenty-three and Sam was twenty-one, and both of them wept before the nuptials took place. People assumed they were crying with joy, but in fact the opposite was true – there were problems between both couples. I was bridesmaid, now aged six, and wore a hideous burgundy dress; Rosco, a beautiful child with golden curls and big blue eyes, was pageboy.

So I managed to survive the madness of my volatile, Northern working-class family, although I was no better at comprehending my dad's mixed messages of devotion and scorn by the age of seven than I had been as a toddler. I took refuge in the consistent love of my mum, clinging to her like a life raft when my dad was particularly harsh towards me.

However, my unusual home life did give me some skills

for negotiating school life. I was more sophisticated than my peers because I had spent so much time around adults, and because my parents were good at speaking their minds with no subtext whatsoever, I had become an expert at dealing with any blunt insults about my size. This was to become a much-needed skill in the playground.

4
Kicking and Punching

9 stone 12 pounds

Everything about me developed fast and early – from the hairs on my head to my chubby toes – so I suppose it was no surprise that I fast-forwarded into puberty before every other girl in my primary-school class. The circumstances were pretty dramatic, though, and left my nephew, Rosco, traumatised for years.

My sister Ella spent her summers in Guernsey, the place where she was born, and the place where her soon to be ex-husband, Tony, lived. I had gone over to visit her with my mum and dad when I was going into the final year of primary school and almost eleven. It was 1988 and Michael Jackson had just completed the UK leg of his 'Bad' tour. We were due to spend a week with Ella and then return to Blackburn. The prospect of helping my mum out in her shop for the remaining few weeks of the summer holidays didn't thrill me at all; I wanted to stay in Guernsey with Rosco and Ella.

It's such a fabulous place, about as different from dreary Blackburn as you can get. There's sea, sand, boats and incredibly clean air, and *everybody* knows each other. The idea of spending the rest of the summer holidays moving between the marina and the many beaches filled with tourists appealed to me no end.

'Please, please, please can I stay with Ella and Rosco and come back to Blackburn with them?' I begged my mum and dad. They were quite happy about it as they got the easy side of the bargain, but Ella took some convincing.

Rosco and I sometimes fought atrociously. We wound each other up, on occasion resorting to kicks and punches, but at the same time we both knew that the holidays would be miserable and lonely if we were stuck by ourselves. My parents and Ella agreed on condition that Rosco and I behaved.

'We promise we'll be really, really good,' Rosco and I chorused.

'Well, if you two start playing up, your feet won't touch the ground,' said Ella.

But of course the moment my mum and dad were safely on their way home to Blackburn, Rosco and I started fighting like cat and dog. We carried on that way until it was time to return home to Blackburn sixteen days later. Poor Ella was beside herself and couldn't wait to get home.

We were travelling back from Guernsey by boat to Weymouth, and then driving home from there. Ella was sitting chatting to Tony, Rosco's father, in his quarters on the boat, and Rosco and I were in a standard cabin several decks up. A squabble between us escalated into yet another fight. We were arguing over who had the right to sleep in the top bunk and there was a rapid exchange of digs and kicks. Suddenly Rosco gave me a sharp push. I fell from the top bunk, hit the floor with a thud and suddenly felt something wet between my legs.

'Oh, God, I've wet myself,' I cried, and shot into the white-tiled bathroom to clean myself up. I pulled down my knickers, expecting to find them damp with pee, and to my horror found a red fluid.

'Blood, BLOOD!' I shrieked to Rosco. 'You little shit, you've made me bleed. Wait till your mum finds out.'

Ten minutes later the blood was still flowing freely. I'd never seen so much of the stuff in my life. 'I'm gonna bleed to death,' I cried.

Rosco trembled on the other side of the bathroom door, not out of fear for my welfare but out of terror for what Ella would do to him when she found out what he'd done to me. My mum hadn't explained anything about periods to me, so I had no idea that the hot, wet trickle making its way down my thighs was anything other than a potentially fatal injury inflicted by Rosco.

I felt around my privates to confirm that was where the blood was coming from and held up my bloodstained hand in horrified triumph. 'Oh, my God, Rosco, what have you done?' I cried. 'You've ruptured something: I'm going to die now.'

Rosco started sobbing. 'Oh, Mik, I'm so sorry. Please don't tell my mum.' He hugged his knees to his chest and started rocking, trying to reconcile himself to the fact that at the ripe old age of seven he had become a murderer.

I kept darting in and out of the bathroom and dabbing away at the blood. 'It won't stop,' I said grimly. 'We better go and find your mum.'

So Rosco in his Spiderman pyjamas and me in my faded white nightie with teddies on it started half running, half hobbling down the corridor in search of my sister Ella.

The wads of toilet paper I'd stuffed into my knickers to catch the blood held me up. Eventually we found Ella and Tony.

Ella couldn't get much sense out of either of us. I was shouting, 'He did this . . .' and Rosco was shouting, 'She did that . . .'

'Ella, Ella, Rosco knocked me off the top bunk and now I'm bleeding to death,' I said dramatically, managing to get my voice to rise above Rosco's whine.

'You're bleeding! Where?' shrieked Ella.

I dropped my head forward so that my ginger hair covered my face like a veil and pointed. 'Between my legs,' I spluttered through my tears.

Ella looked at me in a slightly peculiar way. 'Has Mum talked to you about periods?' she asked.

I shook my head and looked puzzled. Rosco continued to whimper but sensed that he might be off the hook and didn't face spending the rest of his life behind bars after all.

Tony looked as if he wanted the ground to swallow him up. I think at that moment he would have preferred to dive out of the porthole into the icy sea than have to witness all this drama.

Ella explained in a very rudimentary way to me and Rosco that girls of my age started to bleed once a month when the eggs stored inside them that could turn into babies when they were grown-ups were not needed for that purpose.

'You bleed when your body throws the egg away,' she said gently. 'It doesn't mean you're about to die.'

The incident happened on a Sunday and at that time everything closed on Sundays, so there was no chance for

Ella to pop into the nearest shop once the ship docked in Weymouth to buy me a packet of sanitary towels. Instead I had to put up with the indignity of wads of toilet paper stuffed into my knickers until the following morning when the shops opened again. So that was how my periods started. For all I know, Rosco is still having trauma counselling.

That wasn't the only unhappy holiday memory that Ella had of me. The following year we went on a cheap skiing holiday with my extended family. Fisticuffs broke out between Ella and me, even though Ella was asleep at the time. It was in the days before cheap airlines, and my mum calculated that if we hired a ten-seater minibus, took the ferry to Belgium from Portsmouth and then drove through Europe to Germany, we'd save an absolute fortune. We were on the last leg of this interminable journey and had got most of the way through Belgium. It was the middle of the night. Ella was sharing a double seat with Rosco, and I was in a single seat across the aisle. Rosco deliberately kept poking me, preventing me from sleeping and after several threats to do so, in a fit of pique I lifted up my foot complete with heavy Doc Marten boot and instead of hitting Rosco, caught Ella on the shin. Still asleep, she reared up her head like a disturbed slumbering monster and punched me on the nose without even opening her eyes. Then, satisfied that justice had been done, she went back to her previous position.

When we arrived at our skiing destination the following day, there wasn't enough snow to ski on – just sheets of ice with clumps of gravel poking through – so we had to drive on to Austria in pursuit of snow.

As if Ella hadn't suffered enough at my hands, when we finally got to Austria and started skiing, my toggle caught in the ski lift as I tried to get out at the top of the mountain. I blundered into her, knocking her off balance and enraging my dad's brother Laurie far more than Ella in the process. 'Just piss off down that ski slope,' he yelled. 'You're a fucking liability'.

Unfortunately, he didn't know I had never skied on snow before and wasn't sure what to do, but somehow, sobbing the whole time, I found my way to the bottom. My mum went mad with my uncle when she found me, but as usual Dad refused to intervene and fight my corner. I wondered why I got so excited about holidays, because for one reason or another they made me miserable. My dad's failure to stick up for me was the last straw.

There is only one occasion I can remember him defending me and that was when a mean ginger boy called Steven tried to scare me by picking the legs off insects one by one in front of me. I had always hated insects and was duly terrified. I came home tear-stained and told my dad what had happened. He looked indignant and said that he'd deal with it. He went out into the street and found Steven.

'Is it right that you've been ripping the arms and legs off insects and chasing our Mik with them?' he thundered.

Steven nodded his head. 'It was only an insect,' he said.

'Only an insect,' retorted my dad. 'If I ever find you have been doing that again, I'll come and rip your arms and legs off and see how much you like that.'

Steven started crying and ran home to report my dad's threat to his dad, who happened to be a reverend. The reverend came round to complain about my dad threatening Steven, but my dad stuck to his guns and told the reverend that it was wrong for his son to strip the arms and legs off daddy-long-legs so that he could scare me with them. In the end, seeing that my dad was not prepared to apologise, the reverend returned home.

At the time I swelled with pride that my dad was prepared to stick up for me, but afterwards I wondered if my dad had been so vocal not because he was defending me but because he was as usual sticking up for the under-dog and wanted to make sure that justice was done for the daddy-long-legs.

5
Back-Door Calories

11 stone

Throughout my childhood I had learnt that different people wanted and expected me to be different things. Some liked funny, self-deprecating Mikyla; others preferred the quieter, more thoughtful version of me. I had got on very well with the children at my primary school and had a particular rapport with my final-year teacher, Mr Woods, who liked the fact that I fired intelligent questions at him and wouldn't be fobbed off with a childish explanation. Because we had one teacher for everything each year at primary school, I became adept at moulding myself into the person that I thought each teacher wanted me to be. After a while it became very straightforward becoming a year-on-year chameleon. But I was thrown off course at secondary school when I was suddenly presented with ten teachers, all of whom I felt I had to be someone different with. It was an alteration too far for me and for a while I floundered. Life to me was like one long play, and when I walked into a room I needed to know what role I was playing at that moment. If I didn't, I would inevitably fluff my lines. Eventually, though, I adapted to changing my image once an hour instead of once a year.

My mum had been keen to enrol me in the same school that Ella, Sam and Jay had attended. It was a church school and by far the best in the area. But our failure to attend church meant I wasn't considered for a place. My mum even appealed to the local council, desperate for me to have the best possible education. But she got nowhere. My lovely primary-school teacher Mr Woods was keen for me to take the entrance exam to the local private school and felt I was bright enough to get an assisted place, with some of the fees subsidised by the state.

My dad was having none of it, though, and hit the roof. 'If you think anybody's coming round here and rooting through my finances, you can think again. Besides, if you're bright you'll do well anywhere, and I already pay more than enough taxes to cover your education.'

So state school it was – Billinge High School, to be exact. Billinge was one of the roughest schools in Blackburn and had a predominantly Asian intake. I was never one of the cool kids, but looking years older than I did gave me some clout.

My PE teacher, Mrs Orrell, was very fit and trim, and there was no beating about the bush in her world. One time in the first year when I was on my period, I explained to her that for that reason I couldn't have a shower with the other girls. Instead of giving me a quiet, sympathetic nod, she decided to broadcast my menstrual situation.

'Well, girls, it appears we have a woman in our midst. Mikyla won't be able to take a shower along with the rest of you today.'

Everyone giggled. I was the only one who had started my periods at that point and I wanted to disappear behind the nearest locker. She could also be encouraging, though. I was good at netball and she duly praised me for it. She also offered typically wholesome PE-teacher encouragement to me when I took part in running or aerobics. She even allowed me to substitute the vile green gym briefs that were mandatory for a gym skirt. The briefs were just like big knickers – not a good look for anyone above a size 0.

I was often headstrong and defiant at school, and the head teacher regularly phoned up my mum to complain about my conduct. My dad knew nothing of this because he was out at work, but one time he was unexpectedly at home during the day when my mum was out and he picked up a complaining call from the head.

He listened intently and then said sharply, 'Just deck her if she gives you any bother. It's obvious that the softly, softly approach hasn't worked. That's not the way you do things? Well, I'll do it if you can't – I guarantee you won't get any more lip out of her after that.'

Initially I was horrified when I found out what my dad had said, but then I thought that it might not be such a bad thing – Mr Ecton, the head master, had now seen first-hand my dad's take on parenting and he might be a touch more understanding when I stepped out of line.

I was certainly always bigger than my peers at school, but I think that one of the reasons why I was content with my body shape for so long was because my mum just wouldn't accept any adverse comments about me and always tried to head them off before they reached my ears. Whenever I relayed to her a cruel jibe from someone at school about my size she always brushed it aside with a remark like 'They are only saying that because they're envious of your beauty or your success' or 'People who come out with cruel remarks like that have got a problem, and it's not your problem, Mik, it's theirs.' Invariably her words soothed me and shored up my self-esteem whenever it flagged.

Most of the time at school I gave as good as I got. If kids were mean to me, I learnt how to be double mean back in the hope that next time they'd leave me alone.

There were crappy moments like the times when kids would mimic the sweetcorn ad and shout out, 'Green Giant,' or 'Jabba the Hut' to me when I walked down the corridor. Usually I responded with bravado and never let them think that I was affected by what they said. I understood that confronting bullies was the best way to protect myself against further bullying.

'Has someone got a problem?' I'd say. 'Is something bothering you? Is there not enough room for you to walk down the corridor?' At that point the insulter would usually shake his (it was usually a boy) head shamefacedly. 'Well then why don't you just shut up.'

Some days I was genuinely not bothered by these remarks, but at other times I would cringe inwardly and say under my breath, 'Please leave me alone. What have I ever done to you?'

In my first year at Billinge High, age eleven, I was already wearing the biggest size of school-uniform box-pleat skirt, and by the third year had to have my skirts specially made. I knew I was overweight, but I wasn't overweight enough to want to do something about it by depriving myself of the fatty, sugary foods I adored. Whenever Jay came home on leave from the army he commented on my expanding waistline, not because he wanted to be cruel to me, but because he was genuinely horrified, and as a man who could himself have been overweight if he hadn't watched what he ate and exercised vigorously, he wanted me to pull myself back from the brink of obesity.

There were plenty of slim girls at school, but there were plump ones as well, and I didn't spend too much time comparing myself. I was so absorbed in what was going on at school, both in the classroom and out, that if a cutting remark did plunge me into despair, it rarely lasted long because something amusing or positive would come along and distract me.

With my best friends, Sonia and Grace, we planned and plotted as many different kinds of teenage experiments and rebellions as we could. I wish I knew why I started smoking. Until I got hooked it certainly wasn't enjoyable, and the three of us huddling together in the dark over our cigarettes wasn't particularly cool. Nobody pressurised me into trying cigarettes or into maintaining the habit, unless you count the Asian boys who smoked cannabis in the park and who offered to share their stash with us.

By this time I'd started buying alcohol at the off-licence too. Because I looked so much older than I was, I was never once questioned by the staff. I was able to fund this, and my smoking, with a new ruse – I'd worked out how to divest electricity meters of the money put into them. My mum and dad owned and rented out two houses that backed on to our garden. The houses each had meters that took tokens worth £1. I had a key to the meters, and as there was nowhere to log or monitor the number of tokens coming out of the meter, I simply emptied the tokens into a Tupperware box and sold them to the tenants, who came to buy them on a Friday night, only reporting 75% of sales to my parents.

Sonia, Grace and I wore Naf Naf jackets, obtained at a knockdown price from the Asian lads. We modelled ourselves on the Pink Ladies in *Grease*.

The three of us soon moved on to cannabis. I found that it dulled my senses and made me calmer and less hyper-inquisitive at school. I'm sure the teachers found the stoned version of me much easier to manage than the non-chemically altered version. I supplemented my takings from the electricity meters with shoplifting to order. Friends would ask me to procure things like home-perming kits for them. I would steal a £7 kit and sell it to them for £3.

One of the boys at our school was expelled for being disruptive. Being banished from the school wasn't a particularly constructive move for him. He started to fill his days by dealing drugs and often hung around the school gates at 3.30 p.m. to sell to the pupils he knew were consumers.

Sometimes Grace, Sonia and I bought cannabis from him, but we knew he sold other things too. We'd heard about LSD and the magical effects it could have on your mind, and one day Grace and I resolved to try it when we got the chance.

One morning before school we bought one tab costing £3.50 from the school-gates dealer. It was called a 'strawberry triple dip'. The idea had been to save it for the weekend, but on the spur of the moment we decided to swallow it right away. The piece of paper was tiny and we split it in half. At first nothing happened and we wondered if we'd been conned.

'Bet we've been ripped off and it isn't the real thing,' said Grace.

'Yes, trust us to mess it up,' I said.

Throughout assembly and the first lesson neither of us felt a thing. Then we split up into different classes. I had a science lesson and we were working with hydrochloric acid. I spilt some on my fingers and I said to Steven Moores, the boy working next to me, 'Oh, my God, I can't feel my fingers any more. Grace and I dropped some acid this morning and I'm starting to trip. I can see smoke coming out of the test tubes.' Then I started to think about witches and warlocks because of the experiments we were doing. 'Wouldn't it be great if we could all be witches?' I said to Steven.

'Just shut up,' he hissed. 'You're going to get yourself into so much trouble.'

Steven always looked out for me but this situation was beyond his control! Then I began to feel extremely gregarious. When the lesson ended I walked down the corridor to the next one and started going up to almost total strangers and saying, 'Oh, hi, how are you? Nice weather we're having.' People looked at me as if I was mad, but I just carried on. I found Grace sitting down in the middle of the corridor, laughing her head off, her arms and legs flailing like a baby's. At lunchtime Grace decided to throw yoghurt over two girls she didn't like in the schoolyard. She was sent home but I remained in school. The trip was beginning to wear off, although feelings of weirdness kept returning to me in waves.

Outside of my unhealthy experiments with drugs, my

diet was also out of control. By the time I'd been at secondary school for a year or two I had shifted almost imperceptibly from being a big girl to being a fat girl. At that point my mum decided that she should put me on 'diet rations' for my school lunches. Previously she had sent me with uninspiring but edible food – corned beef and pickle or cheese and ham sandwiches.

She devised a concoction almost too horrible to describe – lumpy cottage cheese pinkened with tomato-flavoured pasta sauce. Believe me, there's no food in the world that looks quite as much like sick as that does. It tastes pretty close to it too. I knew my mum had my best interests at heart and I didn't object to her mission to slim me down. It was a preferable approach to my dad's, which consisted of a barrage of insults. He even used to put notes in the biscuit tin to stop me trying to eat too many biscuits. When I surreptitiously opened the tin to grab a handful of my favourite ginger nuts, I often found a note from him saying, 'Piss off, I've counted them.'

'It's good for you, Mik, it'll help you lose a few pounds, and it's tasty too,' my mum reassured me every morning when I peeked at the contents of my lunchbox and pulled a face. I decided that the tomato sauce and cottage cheese combo was either a momentary lapse of sanity on her part or she was getting some kind of percentage from the manufacturers of cottage cheese to force these inhumane substances on me every day. Although I went along with the regime, I devised a cunning plan to acquire the calories my mum was depriving me of. I became a 'rubbish slave' for my friends, who had infinitely more appetising lunches than mine. In exchange for walking across the dining room and putting their discarded food and wrappers in the bin, they were prepared to barter half a sandwich or half a chocolate bar. The most desirable cast-off sandwiches to inherit belonged to my friend Grace. She brought soft-textured brown bread that tasted homemade, smothered in the vegetarian spread Tartex.

My mum had no idea that I had a satisfyingly unhealthy little black-market enterprise going – Mikyla Dodd Back-Door Calories Inc.

I also used to buy other people's sandwiches from them or buy school lunches, or both! One girl, Vereena, was tall, had ginger hair like me but remarkably, unlike me, was extremely skinny. Vereena's parents sent her off to school with healthy sandwiches, but she was desperate to put on weight and so I paid her for her sandwiches and she used the money to buy things like meat and potato pie and chips splashed with gravy. I loved that school dinner too, but not as much as chip teacake with barbecue sauce and a battered sausage from the local chippy. When I got home from school, I ate toast followed by pasta or a jacket potato for tea and sometimes a whole tub of ice cream before I went to bed. What had started out as a healthy appetite as a child had turned to gluttony in my teens.

Whenever he was around Jay remonstrated with my mum about my weight: 'Why do you keep on feeding her, Mum?' he said.

My mum loved me so much that she wasn't very objective about my size. My dad's view, despite the notes in the biscuit tin, was 'If food shuts her up, let her eat.'

My sister Sam rarely commented, obsessed as she was

with shaving a few more pounds off her already skinny frame. Ella also adored me too much to want to hurt my feelings by bringing up the issue.

I did experience cruel jibes from time to time, particularly from my dad: 'Should we unhinge your jaw so we can fit all that in?' or 'I bet you can down that whole plateful in one.' Everyone laughed except me. I was deeply hurt by the insults, but they didn't drive me to a diet of lettuce and grilled chicken. Instead I took refuge in the well-known cycle of the overweight: eat more and more to drown out more and more misery.

Jay tried to incentivise me by offering me £10 for every pound in weight that I lost, and even though his offer was appealing, it didn't work. When he came home on leave, he initiated after-school runs round the park. Because he struggled with his weight but kept things under control, he couldn't see why I couldn't do the same. I could barely run to the end of the road, but he dismissed my protestations as weakness. He urged unfit Ella to do the same. The army had given him a very regimented view of life and Ella's poor health and my excess weight appeared as minor obstacles to him.

'The word "can't" is all in the mind. If you believe you can do it, you will. Now COME ON!'

Doing my best to be the obedient little sister, I ran until my face was so red it looked as if it was going to explode. My breathing turned to gasps and my vision went blurred. Even when we got home there was no respite. Jay insisted on a twenty-minute session of sit-ups, dorsal raises and judo (don't ask).

He was just as pushy with Ella, despite her chronic

asthma. 'Come on, Ella, don't give up now – you can do it.' Ella panted horribly as she struggled round the park and spent the next three days lying on the sofa recovering.

I managed better but hated the enforced 'boot-camp' runs so much that I used to come home and burst into tears in the hope that my mum would take pity on me and convince Jay to release me. She didn't, because although she hated seeing me miserable, she knew that the running would do me good.

I did lose a bit of weight and generally felt healthier, but I didn't have the right mindset. Puffing and panting round the park felt very alien to me. I pretended to have sprained my ankle to get out of a session, and I saw exercise as a justification for eating more than ever, not understanding that that defeated the object entirely.

After my brother returned to Germany where he was stationed, I sometimes went running with my mum. She would sometimes leave me to it and go back to the car and drive to the shop before going home. On one occasion she did just this, leaving me to finish my run in the park. I decided to run to the shop and meet her there instead of going straight home. But by the time I arrived at the shop she had left. I panicked, knowing that when she got home and didn't find me there, she would assume that I'd had my throat slit.

Ella had moved out and was now living not too far from the park, so I sprinted there, thinking I could call my mum from Ella's and put her mind at rest. But when I arrived, Ella was deep in conversation on the phone, and however wildly I gesticulated that I needed to use the phone, she continued talking.

Suddenly a car screeched to a halt outside Ella's house. My dad jumped out, in a rage. I was terrified of what he was going to do to me. I'd never seen him so angry and I was sure that whatever was coming would involve pain. He burst into Ella's house, grabbed me by the scruff of the neck and slammed me against the wall. 'I said I'd bloody kill you when I found you. Do you know how fucking worried we've been?'

I think one reason my dad was particularly angry, apart from concern for me because he had found me at Ella's rather than anywhere else. He resented the amount of time I spent there and knew how much I loved hanging out at her house, dancing together to our favourite music or chatting about the latest bargains to be had at Blackburn Market.

My pleadings with Ella hadn't managed to get her to finish her phone call, but watching my dad laying into me certainly did the trick. 'Sorry, I've got to go,' she said hurriedly. 'Glenn's trying to kill Mik.'

I was still in pain, but I was actually more worried about Ella's beautiful expensive wallpaper than about myself. My dad punched me in the nose and blood spurted everywhere. All I could do was stand there and take it. Thankfully Ella managed to separate us.

My dad emerged from Ella's house in a blaze of anger, saying to my mum, who had been sitting in the car, 'She's here. I told you she bloody would be – that girl is hell bent on causing trouble. She's got to learn.'

My mum jumped out of the car, horrified, I assumed, at the sight of my bloodied face. Instead she made a dash for my jumper and pulled it over my head. I was wearing a Chanel jumper that my mum was very proud of.

'Take that sodding jumper off before you ruin it with all that blood,' she said.

I sat sobbing and wiping little drops of blood in the back of the car. I could see why they were frantic – I had been gone an hour and a half and it was dark by now, and the park was no place for a twelve-year-old – but this reaction was so extreme. With my dad so angry, there was very little my mum could do and in any case I knew she was angry at me too. I was in despair and bewildered by how my plan to give my mum a nice surprise had gone so horribly wrong.

6

If Only We'd Had Sat Nav

15 stone

My dad isn't a bad man, he was just a bad parent to me. Thankfully, during my troubled teenage years my sister Ella was a constant friend. Of my three siblings, she spent the most time with me. All of us adored her. She was without a doubt our family's 'top sister'.

Jay looked up to her because she was his big sister. She was tough and she didn't hesitate to defend him when the need arose. One day at school she marched up to a boy who had hit my brother, said in a steely voice, 'If you touch my brother again, you're dead,' punched him on the nose and then calmly walked off.

She devoted a lot of time to me, and as an attention-seeking child, I loved her even more for taking the time to listen to me chattering away, take me shopping or just chill out with me at her house.

As a teenager, I sought refuge at the houses of other family members, and for me, my cousin Kim and her husband Phil's place was one of the best. Phil was the man I desperately wished could either be my dad or my brother. He laughed at my silly jokes, and although he got along well with my dad, he was perceptive enough to see how much some of the things my dad did hurt me. Phil was a musician and played with various different artists. This work often brought him up to Manchester. He and Kim lived in Harrow, so were ideally located for me to get to Central London, and more importantly they didn't treat me like a child or a hindrance. When I stayed with them, I slotted into their daily routine and talked freely about anything and everything. To keep the cost of travelling to London down, I tried to engineer my visits around any trips Phil had to Manchester and then hitched a ride down to London with him when he'd finished playing with some band or other.

On one occasion Phil was playing with Oasis at Maine Road, Manchester City's ground, so my dad reluctantly agreed to drop me at Phil's hotel after the gig. I said nervously to my dad that I thought I'd be able to direct him to the ground near Rusholme, just south of the city centre. I don't, however, remember volunteering to be my dad's sole guide to Phil's hotel. Well, of course we got lost, and I was an easy target for my dad's fury. After the first couple of nasty snaps from my dad, I decided to call Phil and ask him to direct us. Unfortunately Phil was as clueless as I was. Suddenly, while I was mid-conversation with Phil, my dad butted in, shouting, 'He's from London, you barmy bitch, he won't know. He's just the poor bastard waiting for you to work out where the fuck we are . . . Typical, just fucking typical!'

I sat there cringing. In my left ear, one of my favourite people was speaking calmly and trying to be constructive, while one of my least favourite people was screaming expletives into my other ear. I fought back the tears just long enough to tell Phil I'd call him back. Over the next twenty minutes my dad called me every name under the sun.

'You only care about stuffing your face instead of about important things like directions. You've got Phil waiting to drive you to London so you can empty their fridge and double up as a waste-disposal unit,' he snarled.

He was full of venom and rage, and I genuinely didn't know where it had come from. By the time we drove into the hotel car park I was on the verge of being sick. My stomach was in knots and I was choking on my own tears. To save Phil added embarrassment, I pulled myself together as best I could and got out of the car. My dad greeted him as if nothing had happened. I struggled to get my bag out of the back seat of our hatchback because I was in such a hurry, and right there and then never wanted to lay eyes on my dad ever again. As he pulled away in the car, he shouted feebly, 'Have a good time, Mik.' He was keen to come across as a decent dad in front of Phil, whom he admired. I stared straight ahead. I couldn't bring myself to turn round and look him in the eye.

In Phil's car, I sat with tears rolling down my cheeks staring out of the window. What had I done to make him so angry? I knew I didn't deserve such a tirade of abuse. Why on earth should I have been able to find my way to a strange place in a city I was unfamiliar with when my dad couldn't do that himself?

Phil had sensitively picked up on the situation and for a while he said nothing. Then, in a fatherly manner, he stroked my knee and said gently, 'Just have a good cry – you'll feel better afterwards.'

I took him at his word and burst into noisy sobs. His

kindness amplified my dad's cruelty. Phil was right – I did feel better, and after I'd cried myself out we stopped at a service station and true to form I bought one of everything – a bumper packet of crisps, chocolates, sandwiches and an ice cream, all washed down with the world's favourite diet drink. I don't think I'll ever completely stop reacting that way to distress, but now the impulse to binge away grief is tempered by the thought of how tough it will be to lose the weight afterwards.

At that moment, though, all I cared about was getting the biggest possible sugar rush. For a few moments I was held inside a very pure form of contentment. It was as good as taking any prescription medicine and for years I overdosed regularly. Unlike with a drug overdose, though, I wasn't rushed to A&E but rather, left to get on with it.

During that period I was becoming more and more addicted to junk food. I bought myself teacakes, iced fingers and vanilla slices on my way home from school and continued to illicitly purchase or bribe my way to my friends' school dinners. In a couple of years I had gained almost 4 stone and I was beginning to loathe my expanding body. I had made a few abortive attempts at dieting, but giving up the foods I loved made me grumpy. I couldn't understand how I could get past hunger. As far as I was concerned, it was like getting past death.

After my dad-induced trauma and the subsequent pain relief, I looked at Phil adoringly and thought to myself, I hope I marry a man as kind and understanding as you are.

As with most things in life, though, when he came along, my first love didn't turn out the way I'd dreamt he would be.

7
Am I his Girlfriend?

Flashback – 12 stone

When I was twelve, I looked at least sixteen. I was very developed, which might explain how I found myself, aged twelve, with a sixteen-year-old boyfriend, who became my first lover. In some ways I was very confident and had the self-assurance of someone older. I was able to hold my own in conversations about social issues, religion and even politics. Most of my opinions were based on things I'd heard at dinner parties in my home when any of my peers would have long been dismissed to their beds. I did and still do enjoy lively debate. As a child, I was fascinated by the way people seemed to fearlessly challenge my dad in a way that I never dared to. His views were reactionary and mostly extreme, and he was usually in the minority. Eavesdropping on these challenges reassured me that he was flawed and that his behaviour towards me was just another example of him not seeing things quite the way other people did.

Ninety per cent of the students at Billinge High were Asian. Unsurprisingly, given the demographics, my first boyfriend was Asian. I'll call him Kal, though that's not his real name. He had thick, black curly hair, incredible green

63

eyes and a smile to die for. I'd absolutely set my heart on him. The few white girls at the school were generally very disparaging about the Asian boys, but one of them did grudgingly say to me, 'He may be a Paki but he's actually quite fit.'

For a long time I was too terrified to speak to Kal because I fancied him so much. Even to this day I become so overwhelmed and uncomfortable in the presence of someone I fancy that I clam up or utter something insulting to cover up my nerves. I'm generally not the kind of girl who gets chatted up in bars, partly because I don't look like Kate Moss, and partly because the men who do find me attractive are frightened of me and don't know how to approach me. Even then I felt full of contradictions. If I stood and looked at myself in the mirror, I saw an overweight yet attractive, confident young girl.

This was all well and good until I pitched myself against anybody else. Then I saw myself through what I presumed were the critical eyes of others and felt very inadequate. I knew that a size-10 girl with a flat stomach, slender legs and a cute little arse was far more appealing than I was, and not even my sharp humour and cheeky smile could compensate for my ever-growing wobbly bits.

Despite my feelings of unworthiness, Kal and I finally did get together. One evening I happened to go along to the same youth-club disco as him. He took some ecstasy which made him feel a bit worse for wear and I somehow engineered it that I sat outside with him until he felt better.

I kept on reassuring him that the feeling would pass. I had never tried ecstasy but I managed to bullshit convincingly, and my words seemed to take the edge off his fear. After a while he did start to feel better and he looked at me through new eyes – part of it was probably because he was still off his nut on drugs, but I had calmed him down and helped him come out the other side of his unpleasant feelings. For that moment at least, this was the most wonderful thing another human being could have done for him. I was suddenly conscious that he was looking at me in a way I hadn't seen him look at me before. There was a connection between us like an invisible thread running from his eyes right into mine.

At first our conversation had focused on the effects of the ecstasy on him, but it drifted to other things. In a dreamy way we talked about school, teachers, what music we liked. As we chatted, I started to shiver, and like a true gent he took off his jacket and put it around me. It was a pale blue and white puffa jacket. I was well aware of the significance of a boy giving a girl his jacket, but I wasn't sure if he was giving it to me simply because he could see I was cold or because he wanted to signal that I had become girlfriend material.

I brought his puffa jacket back to school the following day, still uncertain about what it represented. I had been tempted to wash it as it was a bit grubby, but I didn't want to cause offence and I wouldn't have been able to wash and dry it by morning. I agonised to myself that if I hung on to it any longer, he may think I was holding it hostage and making assumptions about him and me that I really shouldn't have been making. So I took it back in its original state and put it discreetly over my arm, not wanting to make a fool of myself by assuming he wanted me to wear it.

My friend Kerris, who fancied him madly, spotted it instantly.

'What are you doing with Kal's jacket?' she said suspiciously. The tone of her voice said loudly and clearly that I couldn't possibly have come by the jacket by legitimate means. 'I'll go and give it back to him,' she said abruptly, full of certainty that either I'd sneaked the jacket when he wasn't looking or that I'd been given it as a result of some terrible misunderstanding. She grabbed the jacket and marched off to find him.

I was upset, but had such a low opinion of my value to any member of the opposite sex that I told myself it was probably for the best, that she was much slimmer and prettier than me so he would be far more interested in her than he would me.

Moments later Kal appeared to challenge me. 'Where's my jacket?' he said already knowing the answer but wanting to hear it from me.

'Oh, Kerris's got it,' I said timidly.

'What's she doing with it?' he said irritably. 'I gave it to you to wear, not to her. Don't do that again.'

I wasn't sure how to respond to that. 'OK,' I said meekly.

The relationship between us was quite peculiar. We never became formal girlfriend and boyfriend the way other people at school were, but we did become good friends and did lots of things together. There were no public displays of affection between us, however. I longed to wander across the school playing field with his arm draped publicly and protectively across my shoulder, making a statement to our peers that I was his and he was mine. I was totally in love with him, and he seemed to love me back, but in terms of our official status together I never knew quite what we were.

We talked about everything under the sun. He opened up to me about his family, his hopes and his dreams. The emotional connection we had was like nothing I'd ever experienced before.

Most of our time was spent in the YMCA or in different nooks and crannies in Blackburn's Corporation Park. That was a great place for romantic interludes during the summer months, but rather bleak and cold throughout the winter.

Corporation Park was where my dad had first made it clear to me in no uncertain terms, that should I even contemplate a relationship with a person of another race I would be severely punished and no longer considered part of the family. 'If I ever catch you with one of those Pakis, I'll nail you both to a tree,' he said. 'And don't forget if you have sex with a Paki, no man will ever want to touch you again.'

Regardless of my dad's repeated warnings – perhaps even because of them – I couldn't stay away from Kal. Now when I look back, although I still don't agree with my dad, I can understand some of his reasoning. Most of the Asian guys my friends and I dated were already betrothed to others in arranged marriages and were merely biding their time with white girls. Of course, I was too young and foolish to heed my dad's warnings and didn't care what happened in the future. I just wanted somebody wonderful to call my own. Kal and I sat on park benches around a beautiful lake and he said over and over again, 'You're amazing, you know.'

I often talked to him about my feelings of inferiority and how there were so many things I simply wasn't capable of doing, but he brushed all my self-doubt aside: 'You can do anything you want to do, you know. You're so beautiful and you're the cleverest person I know. Follow your dreams and be true to yourself.' He appreciated both my physical and emotional maturity: 'All the others in your year are girls, but you're a woman.'

A girl we knew called Linda invited us to a party and we ended up in her bed together. She fell asleep on the floor, and as Kal and I lay there kissing and cuddling, it became clear that he wanted to have sex with me. I didn't know what to do. I knew that twelve was rather young to be embarking on sex. I frantically ran through the options in my head as he got more and more insistent on progressing beyond the kissing and fondling stage that had so far been the physical boundary of our relationship. I thought that if I said no, I'd ruin everything, and absurdly for a twelve-year-old, who was far too young to be doing anything like this, I thought to myself, Maybe this will be the only chance I ever have of experiencing sex. I felt that maybe fat girls would only get offered sex once and a negative response would result in the privilege being permanently revoked.

So I went along with what he wanted. It wasn't a bad experience, as first times so often can be. He was thoughtful, considerate and attentive, and afterwards he held me all night. I lay awake wondering if our relationship had at last become official and if he'd parade me around school as his 'girl'.

But it didn't happen. I didn't see him for a fortnight, and

when I next bumped into him he was very offhand with me. His coolness was as painful as if he'd plunged a dagger right into my heart. Oh, no, what have I done? I've gone and ruined everything by being easy, I wailed to myself.

I plucked up the courage to confront him about his chilly behaviour. 'I want to talk to you about what's happened between us,' I said. 'At the very least you owe me a conversation. I'd rather you were brutally honest about that night at Linda's house than that you just blank me.'

'It was great, it was fun,' he said a little awkwardly.

'So what happens now?' I said.

'Well, nothing,' he replied uncertainly. 'We just carry on.'

'But you're being weird towards me. I haven't seen you for two weeks and I feel like you're avoiding me.'

'I'm feeling a bit confused,' he muttered.

'You're confused,' I said. 'I'm twelve, I'm pretty bloody confused.'

The situation became more and more bizarre. Other opportunities arose to sleep together, which we took, but in public we continued not to be a couple. Then he asked my friend Karen out. She became his official girlfriend, but he wasn't sleeping with her, he was sleeping with me. That was unbearably painful for me, but I was so terrified of Kal ending our relationship if I kicked up a fuss about his official girlfriend that in the end I only mentioned it timidly and didn't pursue it.

I didn't know what to do. I consulted my friends but none of them had had sex or been involved in such a complicated set-up, particularly an inter-racial one with the attendant social taboos. I couldn't talk to my mum, even though I was very close to her, because she would have been absolutely horrified if she'd known I was sleeping with Kal at such a young age. I prayed she'd never find out.

So the unsatisfactory situation continued. News spread at school that I was 'with' Kal in a non-girlfriend sort of way. Some of the teachers got to know too, including one who didn't like the way I answered him back, and sometimes locked me in the storeroom to punish me for some imagined crime. On one of these occasions he shouted to me through the door, 'You're a Paki-loving slag.' These days a remark like that would lead to instant dismissal, but no one seemed to hear him say it except me, and I knew there was no point complaining because it would be a case of my word against his, and my reputation in the staffroom wasn't the best. So instead I just shouted back through the door, 'And you've got small-man syndrome – why don't you leave me alone and go get a job as one of Santa's little helpers instead!' That was one advantage of being tall: they all looked small from where I was standing.

What made the whole Kal situation more taboo was that the Asian and the white pupils rarely hung out together. A kind of apartheid system operated. All the white kids sat together on one 'minority' table, while the Asian kids occupied the rest of the desks. In religious studies we did 50 per cent Islam, 20 per cent between Hinduism and Sikhism and the remainder on Christianity and Judaism – a bizarre ratio for a Church of England school, but it did give me a greater understanding of our multicultural society.

Food became more of a comfort and a companion than ever before during my relationship with Kal. There were so many ups and downs with him and I rarely knew where I stood. In contrast food was always there, dependably waiting for me and never letting me down. Every time I thought my relationship with Kal was over I ate a little bit more because I thought, Well, he's never going to see my body ever again.

Most of my lessons in school were a blur because I was smoking increasing amounts of cannabis. I was sleeping with Kal more regularly and knew enough about birth control to know that he should be using a condom. But every time I mentioned the subject to him he refused to consider it.

'I don't want to use a condom, OK. You're the only person who's never given me grief and now you've started giving me grief,' he said.

At that point I threw a tantrum. Enraged, he slapped me across the face.

'Shut your fucking mouth unless you want another one,' he growled.

I ran home. My mum could see that I was distraught and, ever my protector and defender, was very unhappy that anyone was making me miserable. I gave her a censored version of the truth about Kal. She accepted that I was having a relationship with an Asian boy but assumed it was all quite childish and innocent. It was vital that my dad didn't get to know, though. I couldn't begin to imagine what he would do to me if he found out. Jay was on leave at the time and also got to know about Kal. He vowed to track him down. I begged him not to go after Kal, but he wasn't listening.

'What mosque does he go to, Mik? You've got to tell me

– it's for your own good. I'm not having anybody going around treating my little sister like that.'

'I've no idea which mosque he goes to. Please leave it, Jay – going after him won't help anything.'

In the end, with no leads, Jay called off the Kal hunt.

Later I talked to my mum again about Kal. 'I know you think he's a bastard, but I love him. He's done me so much good. He's encouraged me, given me confidence. When I'm scared of doing things, he urges me on and says, "Go on, you can do it – you're worth ten of them."'

My mum didn't look convinced, but she didn't pursue the matter.

For the next six weeks I didn't see Kal at all. The separation was intolerable. All I could think about was his soft brown skin, his shy smile and his gentle touch. I edited out memories of the slap, the way he didn't want to publicly own up to being with me and the times when he was offhand towards me.

Then I saw him at my friend Grace's house when her father was out. I looked at him and he looked at me. Without uttering a word, both of us said with our expressions how much we'd missed each other. We disappeared upstairs into Grace's bedroom and didn't return until minutes before her dad returned home.

During the highs and lows of my relationship with Kal, I became very close to my music teacher, Mrs Pate. Like me, she was overweight and very direct. There was an instant affinity between us. She encouraged me, was very fond of me and wasn't intimidated by my opinionated nature. In fact she enjoyed and even encouraged it.

Other teachers would tell me how fiercely she defended me when I was the subject of dissatisfaction in the staffroom. I had a part in the school play in which she was chief organiser. I was Mrs Potiphar in *Joseph and the Amazing Technicolor Dreamcoat*.

I applied myself when I hadn't seen Kal for a while, but one weekend when we met up I was very distracted during rehearsals at school the following day.

Afterwards Mrs Pate took me aside. 'Have you been seeing that boy Kal?' she said.

'Yes,' I said quietly.

'And?'

'I slept with him,' I said, hanging my head.

She looked worried. 'Did you use any protection?'

I shook my head. I knew that she had my best interests at heart, but I was squirming under the glare of her scrutiny.

'Right, here's ten pounds. Go down to the chemist's, buy yourself a pregnancy testing kit, do the test and report back to me immediately. If you're old enough to have unprotected sex, you're old enough to face the consequences.'

I did the test at my friend Zoë's house. The whole thing was deeply alien to me. We pored over the instructions, trying to work out what colour line we were supposed to be looking for. When a decisive blue line appeared in the window of the testing stick, Zoë and I gasped together.

'Oh, my God, Zoë, what am I going to do? I'm only thirteen: my dad will kill me, either before or after he kills Kal.' I burst into tears. I knew that I wasn't really old enough to be having sex, and at that moment I felt far too young to deal with the consequences of it.

Zoë was no comfort at all. 'I'm so glad I'm still a virgin,' she said. 'I'm going to keep my legs firmly crossed for ever more.'

I wandered back to school in shock. I knew I had to tell Mrs Pate.

'Well?' she said, knowing the answer before I opened my mouth as she stared at my tear-stained face. She looked at me gravely. 'Oh, dear – try not to upset yourself too much. Leave it with me and we'll get you the right help.'

My trust in Mrs Pate stopped me from sinking into total and utter despair. What I didn't know was that she had a legal obligation to tell my mother about it all.

When I returned home that evening in a daze, I received a call from a friend who asked me why my mum had been at our school that afternoon. Of course I put two and two together and knew my horrifying secret was probably already in my mother's lap.

I sat in my bedroom aimlessly tidying my knicker drawer for lack of anything better to do to occupy my very confused mind. I folded my knickers into perfect squares in the way that someone with serious mental-health problems might do. I dreaded the sound of my mum's key turning in the lock. She arrived home at her usual time and climbed the stairs to my bedroom. I thought I could hear a sighing sound in her footsteps. I couldn't bear to look at her as she walked into my bedroom.

'I'm disgusted with you, you little slut,' she said, her voice quivering as she tried to control her rage and disappointment.

I sat on my bed and wept and said nothing. To make the situation worse, my mum had only a few weeks until she buried her own mother, our beloved nan, so my timing was truly dreadful. I know my mum was shocked that I was having sex, but she hardly had time to process that information because she had to deal with the bombshell about me being pregnant and work out a way to keep the news from my dad – as well as help me plan what to do.

Next I had to tell Kal. I called him and told him I needed to see him urgently. We agreed to meet at the YMCA.

'Kal, I'm pregnant,' I said flatly. I had emptied out all my tears and was very calm.

'What the fuck are you telling me for?' he said.

'Because it's yours,' I replied.

'What do you want me to do about it? What do you want me to say?' he said helplessly.

'Well, have you got any suggestions?'

'I don't know – buy a knife and cut it out,' he said coldly.

'Go fuck yourself,' I shouted. I couldn't believe that he could be so cruel and heartless in the midst of my abject despair. I started sobbing again. 'I slept with you because I wanted someone to love me, to find me attractive and sexy and now I'm paying the price.'

I walked off, becoming increasingly desperate to separate myself from this situation, wondering if it was possible to wish away this feeling. If I concentrated really hard, maybe even talking to the God I wasn't sure I believed in, I could remove this tiny baby from the inside of my womb and give it to somebody who wanted it.

I got cravings early on and typically they were calorific ones. Industrial quantities of butterscotch and at least two vanilla slices a day. I interpreted them as cravings but perhaps I was comfort-eating. Despite whatever drove me to gorge myself on those foods during the early weeks of my pregnancy, I have never touched them since.

I had started to feel terribly sick in the mornings. I was sharing a double bed with my sister Sam at the time, as she was afraid of a supernatural visit from our recently-departed nan. At first she didn't suspect anything when I dived into the bathroom and bolted the door each morning, but after a couple of weeks she cottoned on and asked me outright, 'Are you pregnant?' What could I say? I'd promised my mum not to breathe a word, but I was desperate for somebody to talk to. I told her everything and swore her to secrecy.

A few days later Kal turned up at school when I was on my way home. He looked crushed and remorseful.

'Let me carry your bag,' he said humbly.

I wasn't in the mood for apologies. 'I'm pregnant, not crippled. I'm perfectly capable of carrying my own bag, thank you,' I said coldly.

'What I did was so wrong. I was just scared – I'm still a little boy inside,' he said. 'You're one of the most precious people in the world to me.'

I wasn't prepared to soften. 'Don't worry, I'm not keeping it,' I barked. I could see the enormous relief flooding through his veins.

'OK, it's your decision,' he said, trying to sound casual.

Kal's brother, who had always disliked me, got to know about the pregnancy and decided this was his moment to get one over on me. He wrote a letter to my parents pretending to be Kal's father. He wrote, 'Dear Mr Dodd, that bastard child your daughter is carrying is not my son's: he's a good Muslim.'

Unlike the numerous letters received from my school over the years, we weren't expecting this one, so my mum was unable to intercept it as it fell on to our mat. My dad had returned to bed with the pile of mail so it was a good ten minutes before he actually opened this malicious attempt to ruin my already chaotic life. He came down the stairs like a tornado, with my stunned mum trailing behind trying to work out why this letter had sent my dad to La La Land. He dragged me out of my bed by my hair and onto the landing, where we collided with my mum and sister.

'Is this true? Are you pregnant by some Paki?' he yelled. I was literally petrified. The only thing that was moving were the tears streaming down my face. Still holding on to my hair, he pulled my face close to his and in his most threatening tone he slowly asked, 'Are . . . you . . . PREGNANT?'

I couldn't think my way out of this one fast enough. I just kept sobbing and gasping for air. I was flooded with relief when my mum jumped in.

'Don't be ridiculous, Glenn, I would know if she was pregnant.'

Following my mum's lead, I managed to whimper, 'He's just my friend, I swear.'

My dad wasn't sure whether to believe my mum and me or not. But he decided that even if we were telling the truth, I would be punished for my friendship with Kal by being put under full house arrest. I was banned from setting foot outside the door unless I was going to school and back.

A week or two after my mum found out I was pregnant, she was due to go to Andorra. She asked my music teacher,

Mrs Pate, to take me to our GP and discuss my options. I knew as soon as I saw the blue line on the pregnancy test that I wanted an abortion. My GP was a good, God-fearing Irishman but never once did he allow that to cloud his judgement or challenge my decision. He did strongly suggest I see a counsellor, but I rejected the offer. I had made up my mind. I was still a child myself and I didn't want to be responsible for another one. I was determined to succeed and get what I wanted from life and knew that I'd make a lousy parent in these circumstances.

When my mum got back from Andorra, we concocted a story that would enable me to be absent overnight in order to have the termination. At 8 a.m. she dropped me off at the hospital in my school uniform, stayed long enough to sign a consent form to allow the doctor to perform the procedure, then dashed off to work.

I had no idea what to expect on the ward. There were women in the hospital who had been admitted for a range of gynaecological procedures.

The women in the next bed called across to me, 'What are you in for, love?'

'Abortion,' I said.

She looked sad.

'How about you?'

'I've got polycystic ovaries. I'm trying to get them sorted out so I can get pregnant.' She looked away. I prayed that a hole would open up in the middle of my bed that I could crawl into.

I don't think I've ever experienced a feeling like it. Unlike normal loneliness, where you feel alone and wish somebody was with you, I didn't even feel I was there myself. It was like an out-of-body experience. The real me was unable to speak or feel. I was totally detached, as though this was happening to somebody else.

I couldn't stop thinking about my conversation with Kal the night before. He did a sudden emotional about-turn and pleaded with me not to go through with the termination. 'Please don't kill our baby. Let's try to make it work. We could get married and you could convert to Islam.'

Every time the word 'Islam' was mentioned I knew I was doing the right thing having the abortion. I know I wanted to be an actress, but to pretend to be a Muslim every day for the rest of my life was a bridge too far. Impossible!

The nurses weren't particularly nice to me. They carried out their pre-operative checks with pursed lips. I was glad to drift into the oblivion of the anaesthetic.

I came round feeling horribly sick. I felt empty but in so many ways relieved. Relieved that my soul had re-entered my body. Relieved that I'd survived the operation. Most of all, relieved that I could resume being a teenager with all my dreams and aspirations still a possibility. My mum picked me up the next morning. Like the nurses, her lips were pursed.

We got into the car, and after a couple of minutes she said, 'I don't care what you do, but don't ever lie to me again. The worst thing is not that you got pregnant by some disgusting boy but that I had to find out about it from a complete stranger.'

I vowed that I'd never lie to her again and I never have.

My relationship with Kal carried on after the abortion.

He seemed more devastated than I was about it. Then his parents sent him to Pakistan to get married. I sobbed and sobbed when Kal left. I had developed Bell's palsy, a paralysis of the face, fortunately a mild version in my case, and half of my face had dropped so I could only sob out of one eye. It wasn't quite the sad, dignified, beautiful image I had hoped Kal would have of me for our final parting. He wrote to me regularly from Pakistan, and I rushed downstairs every morning so that I could get my hands on the post before my dad did. If he had seen me receiving letters from Pakistan, he would have gone ballistic.

Several months later Kal returned, having got married, but his wife was going to join him in the UK later. He begged me to continue our relationship. I held out for as long as I could: 'Kal, you're a married man – we can't carry on with this.' But he started climbing up the drainpipe to my bedroom window at night and in the end I relented and let him into my bedroom and my bed. He spent the whole night with me, but when it was time for us to sleep he slept on the floor between my bed and the window so that if by any chance my dad barged in, Kal would be concealed from view. We fell asleep holding hands, my hand dangling over the side of the bed into his.

Our relationship was less passionate than in the early days but more companionable. When Kal's new wife came over from Pakistan, I told him that things between us really had to end now. My dad's words rang in my ears: 'Those Asian men only use white girls to practise on. They always end up marrying one of their own.'

'But my wife would never say anything about our relationship,' he protested.

'That's not the point – we just can't carry on like this. I don't want to become your mistress when I was here first. If you care about me, you'll let me go.'

But Kal wouldn't take no for an answer.

I was still totally in love with him, but I also had a strong sense of self-preservation and I knew that continuing the relationship in these conditions would end up destroying me and would possibly destroy Kal's marriage too. While I loved him as much as ever, the relationship was getting increasingly messy and complicated. It was very stressful keeping it hidden from not only my dad but my friends and Kal's friends and family. I craved a simpler life with no secrets and no deception. I tried to explain this to him, but he was adamant that we could secretly carry on.

In the end, in desperation, I went round to his friend's house and told his friend to tell Kal not to come to my house again. White people didn't generally go to the Asian neighbourhoods in Blackburn, so when I turned up there it created shockwaves in the community. His mother called out to him, panicked, 'Come, come, there's a white girl at the door to see you.'

He came outside and we spoke in the middle of the street.

'What the hell are you doing here?' he said.

I stood there sobbing and said, 'You've got to make Kal understand that he can't come round to my house any more. If he turns up again, I'll have to come round here and embarrass you again.'

Kal never clambered up my drainpipe again. I loved

him still and I knew he loved me, my soul and my entire being. It had been a complicated first love, often a troubled one, but also a love that had made my heart soar.

8
'Lena's Come Home'

15–16 stone

Academically, I did fairly well at school. I was in a lot of the top sets and remained there throughout my school career, much to the dismay of many of my teachers. I was a difficult pupil, always asking questions and challenging them to quantify any grey areas. I think I wanted to know what they thought as people, rather than being satisfied with what the books said. I was copying behaviour at home, where people shouted different opinions over each other until somebody conceded. I listened carefully and soaked up these arguments like a sponge. It made me feel that I needed to hear at least two opinions on every subject in order to form my own view.

Looking back, I think my very vocal behaviour in the classroom was a way to distract people from my obvious problem with food. While teachers focused on how mouthy I was, I could continue overeating in peace.

While many of the teachers found my wilfulness challenging, Mrs Pate welcomed my spirited contributions. She recognised that I had a bright, inquiring mind and wanted to feed it. She arranged a trip to *Les Misérables* at the Palace Theatre in Manchester for some of the older students but said I could go along too if my mum gave her permission. My mum did, and I had an absolutely magical evening. I understood the messages in the production. I sobbed and sobbed at the heartbreaking plot and vowed to save up to buy a tape of the show. When I did, I listened to it over and over again. I implored my very busy mum to listen and one day she agreed. She, too, was smitten, although she had to wait a year and a half before the production came back to Manchester.

Going to the theatre and becoming totally entranced in the dramatic storyline of *Les Misérables* and the way the actors and the stage sets brought this period in the distant past totally to life was revelatory to me. The only shows I had been to before were pantomimes, which, while fun and entertaining, were not in any way comparable with this experience. Seeing theatre at its best was a pivotal moment for me. I envied the actors, who looked as if they were having such a fabulous time inhabiting the skin of imaginary human beings. I had always loved entertaining my friends and family with jokes and anecdotes, and suddenly acting seemed to me like a logical progression. I left the show excited, not only about the power of what I had just seen but beginning to dream that this was something I might be able to do with my life.

In my second year my school staged a production of *Bugsy Malone*. I enthusiastically auditioned and was given the fairly small part of Lena Marelli, a loud, blousy woman. At first I was disappointed not to have been given a bigger role, but I soon learnt that it was the quality of the role and the lines that counted, rather than the quantity.

I made a dramatic entrance from the back of the room in

a long, sequinned dress and a flamboyant ankle-length fur coat. As I walked down the central aisle towards the stage, all eyes turned in my direction. I knew from the way everybody looked at me and laughed that I had made an impression on what had been until then a fairly bland and typical school production. Although I was only twelve, I was probably about 5 foot 9 inches tall at the time and weighed about 12 stone. I could easily have passed for a sixteen year-old. I had to shout out to a slim blonde member of the cast, 'OK honey, beat it back to Iowa. This show has got its star back. Lena's come home.'

I was hooked on the adrenaline buzz of performance. Afterwards several of the teachers hurried up to my mum and enthused, 'Wasn't she amazing?'

My mum says that that was the first time she thought that I had talent. But while some of the teachers encouraged me, others tried to crush my enthusiasm, not just because I was tall, fat or ginger, but because I was a working class girl from Blackburn and shouldn't be getting ideas above my station about fame and fortune.

My brother, Jay, also tried to put a damper on my fledgling thespian ambitions: 'No one wants to see a fat person on the telly,' he said.

My mum, of course, didn't share these views. Keen to nurture my burgeoning interest in drama, she found out about something called Oldham Theatre Workshop and put my name down for it when I was in year nine, aged thirteen. I heard nothing and more or less forgot about it. I consoled myself that I could continue acting in the annual school play. I had ambitions to land a starring role by the time I got to year ten. I felt I had proved myself with my apprenticeship in more minor roles in the first two years. In year ten, the show selected was *Oliver* and I had set my heart on being Nancy. I was a big personality like Nancy, and I was absolutely convinced that this was a role with my name on it. I was certain that I would get the part, and when my teachers announced that the role had gone to another girl, I was distraught. I felt as if my entire world had come crashing down around my ears. I had planned everything around getting the role of Nancy.

But in my life bad has a habit of being followed by good, and like manna from heaven a letter plopped on to the doormat a couple of days later that banished my gloom in seconds.

It was a letter from Oldham Theatre Workshop inviting me to take up a course there. I knew that the workshop had an excellent reputation and had spawned a whole host of stars on soaps like *Coronation Street* and *Brookside*.

I literally jumped for joy when I read the letter. Nothing could have healed the pain of failing to get the Nancy part as effectively as this did. Had I got the part of Nancy in the school play, I wouldn't have had time to accept the offer of Oldham Theatre Workshop. Everything had worked out for the best. Because school productions were always musicals, I had thought of singing and acting as two interlocking disciplines that couldn't be separated. Once I got into thinking in theatre-workshop mode rather than school-play mode, I realised that being an accomplished singer wasn't the be all and end all. I decided to focus on becoming a proper thespian.

I was very apprehensive the first time I went to the workshop. I was fourteen and assumed that the standard of acting would be incredibly high and that my amateur efforts would stick out like the sorest of thumbs as soon as I opened my mouth. The workshop was very close to the town centre. It didn't look particularly salubrious, and was accessed via a dark alley that led to a narrow cobbled street. On a rickety little door was a barely legible sign, which read, 'Oldham Theatre Workshop.'

'Are you sure this is it?' I asked my mum doubtfully. I had imagined something much grander.

'Well, the sign says so,' said my mum.

Inside, the floors were cold stone covered with black paint as thick as tar. We walked up a flight of stairs and found our way to the big hall. Blackburn wasn't an especially exciting place to live, but as soon as I stepped inside Oldham Theatre Workshop I felt a ripple in my soul. I didn't know how exactly, but I knew that things were going to change in my life.

Oldham Theatre Workshop was run by David Johnson. He had an impressive reputation and ran the workshop as a benevolent dictatorship. There was no board or panel to seek redress from if you weren't happy with the role David had handed out to you. David Johnson *was* Oldham Theatre Workshop. He was a kind man but also a tough task master. As far as he was concerned, talent was of no use to him unless it was accompanied by steely discipline. There was no space for fledgling prima donnas on his watch. When people went for auditions and said that they'd trained with David Johnson at Oldham Theatre Workshop, casting directors knew that at the very least the actor would show up on time with all their lines learnt.

The first time I saw David, he didn't walk into the room,

he made an entrance. I wondered if that was something for the benefit of newcomers like me, but in fact he did the same thing every time I saw him. He always dressed in a navy-blue shirt, black trousers and black slip-on leather loafers. His hair was thick and black and looked like a wig, although it wasn't. He had podgy fingers and short legs. When I saw him, I couldn't take my eyes off him. He had a certain aura. He had been an actor many years ago but had then gone into directing and found his niche there.

At school I was often cheeky to my teachers, obeying their instructions only if I liked them. With David Johnson it was different. I obeyed him because I feared him. After my dad he was only other person I'd been scared of in my life.

Actors who turned up late for rehearsals or spoke when he was speaking were quite simply dismissed from his workshop. I worked as I'd never worked before under David's instruction. I'd tasted rejection with the Nancy part and I didn't like it. I vowed that my work at Oldham Theatre Workshop would be exemplary at all times so that rejection would simply not be a possibility. I was totally at peace now with not getting the role of Nancy. In my mind everything was sorted.

I had secured the very unglamorous role of a cow in extracts from *Animal Farm* at Oldham Theatre Workshop. I hadn't read George Orwell's *Animal Farm* at that point and so did not fully appreciate the significance of my one and only line: 'I haven't been milked for a week, moo.'

We were rehearsing for a special show to mark twenty-five years of the workshop, which included highlights from some of the most successful previous shows. One of the most blissful things for me about being involved in the workshop was that David treated me like a 'normal' girl. My weight wasn't an issue for him and was seldom referred to. All that interested him was whether I could act or not. To me, David was God.

However, he was clear that although he thought I was a good actress that with my height, weight and hair colour I was not castable at the moment but would be as a character actress in the future. I was perfectly happy with this analysis. I knew that if I was being cast for *Romeo and Juliet*, I would always be the nurse and not Juliet. I tried to see the positive in everything, and instead of descending into a deep depression because I would never be selected for Sharon Stone-style roles, I decided that it was a good thing that I was going to be a character actress, not just relying on stereotypical good looks to get me roles. As a character actress, I knew that I may be able to get more challenging roles and would be forced to have more strings to my bow than I might if I looked conventionally beautiful.

The anniversary show we were working on contained a medley of extracts from different books and plays. Several narrators were required and I was thrilled to be chosen as one of them. My policy was to volunteer for every part going. David was also looking for people to take part in the finale. Of course my hand shot up, although perhaps I would have hesitated rather more had I known the costume we were all expected to wear – a black leotard, fishnet tights, a silver, spangly waistcoat and a bowler hat – not my best look! But once I had volunteered, it was difficult to back out. Getting hold of a pair of fishnet tights that would fit a 6-foot, 15-stone girl was no easy feat. My mum, as ever, came up trumps and tracked down a pair. They cost her £19.50, which is a lot these days and was even more thirteen years ago. She instructed me to avoid laddering this precious piece of clothing on pain of death.

Although my body was on show as never before, it didn't curb my growing appetite for junk food. I still adored burgers and chips but also developed a taste for Cantonese chicken and fried rice. Ella and I made a beeline for big strawberry tarts filled with creamy custard, drizzled with strawberry syrup and piled high with cream. I indulged my appetite for whatever took my fancy.

It was at Oldham Theatre Workshop that I met Suranne Jones for the first time. She was tall and very pretty with womanly curves and had lots of boys after her. We didn't start off well together. Her real name was Sarah Jones, but for her equity card she needed to have a unique name so she took her grandmother's name Suranne. I felt intimidated by her – she was popular, vivacious and could sing, dance and act. I felt as if she was a threat to the fragile but growing sense of security I was gaining at the workshop. I convinced myself that she was ignoring me. Shortly after, though, in 1992, we were filming an advert to promote the UK's bid for the 2000 Olympics and we became firm friends. The advert involved lots of children releasing balloons. There was a woman involved in the workshop who had had polio as a child and who was slightly disabled as a result. She wasn't a particularly nice woman and scoffed at the suggestion that she should be in the advert. Suranne was supposed to say, 'You can leap in front of the camera,' but instead she accidentally said, 'You can limp in front of the camera.' She and I dissolved into fits of giggles. Fortunately David wasn't there to see it.

Once we got to know each other, I discovered that her life wasn't as perfect as I had assumed it to be. Although she seemed very confident, she had been badly bullied at school and was a bit insecure about her appearance, like most teenagers, because she wasn't super-skinny like some of the other girls. She became one of my closest friends and I made a mental note to myself to try not to make such snap judgements about people in the future. Later on, when I landed my part in *Hollyoaks*, she was delighted for me. Three months after that she got the part of Karen McDonald in *Coronation Street* and of course I was delighted for her. We've been friends for fourteen years now and in the world of TV, which is disproportionately populated by shallow, grasping people, it is a joy to spend time with someone who has always been so honest and genuine.

After the Oldham Theatre Workshop anniversary production I got a part as a fairy in the Christmas pantomime *Snow White and the Seven Dwarves*. I was thrilled, although the gaudy orange material out of which my mum was supposed to fashion a costume for me was not flattering.

Lisa Riley was also in the pantomime and was working as an actress. I was very envious because I was dying to get a paid job. I was conscious when I worked with Lisa that there was only so much room for a pretty, funny, fat girl and that we were unlikely to both land a plum role. I also knew that Lisa had been working for longer than me and was ahead in the pecking order. She played the funny Buttons character.

In fact that particular panto was full of actors who went on to become soap regulars. Along with Lisa and Suranne, who played Snow White, there was Anthony Cotton, who now plays Sean Tully in *Coronation Street*, and two of the dwarves were played by Cleveland Campbell and Kelvin Fletcher, who went on to play Danny Daggert and Andy Sugden in *Emmerdale*.

There are many others who attended Oldham Theatre Workshop and went on to become household names. David used to say to us, 'Turn on the TV any night of the week and I challenge you not to be able to find one of my ex-pupils.'

I still do that and have yet to prove him wrong. It's hard to put into words what a wonderful experience the work-shop was for all of us. The atmosphere was amazing, and we were all so hungry for success.

The panto run lasted for two months, and it fell to my dad to chauffeur me back and forth between Oldham and Blackburn. There was seldom conversation on the journey but I was grateful for his contribution. Rather than coming in to watch me perform the same thing over and over again, he took himself off to the local cinema and watched *Cliffhanger* with Sylvester Stallone over and over again. Sometimes he would be forced to just wait patiently in the car with a flask of coffee.

Although Suranne had the lead role in the panto, she ignored the acting pecking order of only fraternising with other lead actors. Instead she mucked in with people like me from the plebeian class. I remember one of the leads walking over to Suranne and trying to persuade her to join the other leads in the 'prini (principles') corner', as it was known. This was an area sectioned off with runner rails to keep the riff raff out. I was over the moon when she politely but firmly declined the offer.

The eight-week run of the panto was exhausting and involved a lot of adrenaline. Somehow I managed to perform every night, attend school every day and endure the long commute from Blackburn to Oldham. Suranne and I really bonded over that panto, and we bought each other a vanity case, something that a lot of the girls at the theatre workshop had. One of the other girls had a more upmarket Elizabeth Arden vanity case, and one time when she saw Suranne and I admiring our more lowly cases, made a catty remark, 'Oh, Christmas presents, I hope you said a big thank you.'

We ended the panto on a high. To the audience, pantos always look like enormous fun. Often they're just as much fun to rehearse and perform in as to watch. During the run of *Snow White and the Seven Dwarves* we all had an absolute ball.

At the end of the panto David said that he had picked out sixteen people to work on an Easter play. To our delight, both Suranne and I had been chosen. But tragically it was not to be.

Over the years the education department at Oldham County Council had become more and more involved with the work of the theatre group and made an increasing number of demands on David to abide by various council protocols. David kicked against the ever-growing quantity of bureaucratic rules and regulations imposed on him. 'I'm not a social worker or an accountant, I'm a creative director,' he exploded.

Apparently, out of nowhere, a vicious whispering campaign began about David. False rumours circulated about him. In the end the pressure became intolerable for him and he withdrew from the theatre group.

David was very popular with all of us and we felt devastated for him that he had been pushed out by a campaign founded on cruel and baseless rumours because he wouldn't conform. For us, the workshop was a lifeline. I was pretty sure my dad would never agree to send me to drama school and this was my best hope of carving out an acting career for myself. Another of the teachers from the workshop set up an improvisation-based project, but it just wasn't the same as when David was in charge.

I was at a loss as to what to do next, but about a couple of years later, when I was finishing school, something wonderful happened. I heard that David had set up a new theatre group. I was nervous of seeing him again after his breakdown in case he was terribly diminished. He had found part of an old building in the centre of Manchester to rent. As I sat waiting and wondering what sort of state David would be in, he appeared and greeted me effusively.

'Hello, Mikyla. It's absolutely wonderful to see you.' He hugged me and seemed quite excited. 'How are you? Apparently quite a lot of the old school are coming. We'll really be able to have a blast.'

As more and more of David's faithful disciples gathered, he started talking about the kinds of things we'd be doing – Shakespeare and Restoration plays were on the agenda, much more adventurous material than we'd tackled at Oldham Theatre Workshop.

When he'd finished briefing us, he beamed. 'May I say to all of you thank you very much for coming. It's delightful to see old faces and new.' He seemed more humble and more human than when I'd first met him. He still had a Benny Hill kind of chubbiness. Apparently he had lost a lot of weight after his breakdown but he had put most of it back on again by the time I saw him. My acting career was on track again. I was euphoric.

9
Finding a New Comfort Zone

17 stone 7 pounds

I wore very unflattering clothes in my teenage years – shapeless, elasticated jeans, baggy tee-shirts and, horror of horrors, floral skirts with indeterminate waistlines. I assumed that there were no other options available. One day while I was still at school my mum decided to take me shopping to Blackpool. I stumbled upon an Evans shop – known then as Evans Outsize.

'What's this?' I said, suddenly sensing that there was another clothing life out there just waiting to be discovered.

My mum looked rather disinterested. She had been reluctant to reveal to me the existence of such places because she felt it would give me licence to eat even more, knowing that I would still be able to buy fashionable clothes. She hoped that if my only options were baggy, shapeless, drab clothes, that it might spur me on to lose weight to fit into things which were more appealing.

'It's a shop which caters for bigger sizes,' she said sheepishly.

'Why didn't you tell me before?' I whooped. 'Let's go inside. At last I'll be able to look halfway decent.'

It was an even better feeling than wandering into Santa's

grotto as a child and knowing that at least some of the presents piled up around Santa's ankles would be for me. At the time I was a size 18-20. My eyes widened when I saw that sizes up to 32 hung on rails. I bought a beautiful cream, embroidered shirt in a size 30-32.

'Er Mik, I don't think you need such a big size,' said my mum.

'Mum I'm buying it in this size because I can. That's such a thrill to me.'

I got chatting to the woman who ran the shop. She asked where I was from and when I said Blackburn she said: 'Oh, we've got a store in Blackburn too you know, might be a bit nearer for you, we're all over the place.'

My mouth kept dropping open in amazement at finding a shop which made eye catching, flattering fashionable clothes for thousands of girls and women just like me.

On returning to Blackburn I made a point of finding Evans. On my first visit I struck up an instant rapport with the manager, Karen.

'Do you have a job?' she asked.

'No, I'm still at school.'

'How about a Saturday job?'

'No I don't have one.'

'Would you like one? We always need people.'

'Yes I would,' I said eagerly. She got me to fill out an application form on the spot and so my career in retail began.

As I've said, the bad things that have happened in my life have been followed by something good. When I'm in the middle of something unpleasant, I try to hold on to the fact that something good is going to come next. I'm a very strong and practical person. I'm rarely pessimistic and would describe myself as a realistic optimist. This optimism would get me through the tricky period after leaving school.

Because education and I hadn't seen eye to eye, I decided to leave school at the first available opportunity. I got four Bs, one C, three Fs and a U (for my IT) in my GCSEs. I applied for sixth-form college and planned to study drama, psychology and English literature at A level. Psychology particularly appealed to me because I was interested in people, the same interest that made me love acting. Drama school wasn't an option at the time because of the fees, but I was hopeful that with David's drama group and with sixth-form college, I could still go for parts and develop as an actor.

Throughout this time I was working at Evans part-time. I became a firm favourite with the customers, always smiling and ready to help. I was at my best in the fitting rooms, giving advice and offering more flattering alternatives. I enjoyed the atmosphere as we had a very loyal customer base who, at the time, had poor options where clothes shopping was concerned. My quest to slim down was probably not helped by working in an environment populated by overweight female shoppers and overweight assistants. Most of the staff were overweight, so our diet efforts were collective. This meant that if one fell off the wagon, we all tumbled like dominos.

What I noticed after a while was that the women I worked with were already married and settled with a man who accepted them. I was yet to find somebody, and the bigger I got, the less likely it was that that would happen –

not because there aren't men who find heavier women incredibly sexy, but because my dislike for myself intensified the heavier I got, and I didn't want to contemplate another human being seeing me naked. I made feeble attempts to diet while I was at Evans. I tried to limit myself to a couple of ham rolls and a tub of coleslaw during the day, but in the evening when I sat in front of the TV at home, I invariably consumed a huge tub of praline and cream ice cream. Because I was surrounded by big women, I was able to avoid thinking about the fact that my weight was creeping up. I tried not to look at myself in the shop mirrors and bought clothes in one colour only – black.

One thing that did bother me at Evans was that certain customers felt that because they had less-than-perfect bodies, it gave them carte blanche to comment on mine. People assumed that I must have given birth at least once and that I couldn't possibly be the size I was unless it could be explained away as the after-effects of pregnancy.

When people asked me if I had children, I gave them a hard stare and said, 'No.'

'Oh, I see. I just wondered if that was the reason you're overweight.'

I tried to remain calm and collected and asked, 'Do you think if I'd had a baby it would be acceptable to be fat?'

'Er, yes . . . no . . . whatever,' they said, squirming and stuttering.

Others, often the older generation, looked at me sadly and said, 'It's such a shame – you've got a really bonny face.'

'What's such a shame?' I asked, mock naïvely, making them feel profoundly uncomfortable.

Unfortunately making them feel awkward didn't make

me feel any better. People seemed happy enough to make offensive remarks about fatness, yet would never dare address equivalent insults to black or disabled people about the colour of their skin or the fact that they were sitting in a wheelchair. Respect for difference simply didn't extend to surplus flesh.

Although I was mistress of the cutting putdown where 'fatist' remarks were concerned, I remained self-conscious about my size and tried my best to hide it from the outside world.

At college, as part of the drama course, we were expected to attend dance classes, which I didn't look forward to because of my size. I tried to forget the fact that I was expected to attend the lesson and hoped I'd be able to dodge it. Instead I bumped into the teacher, who decided to walk me to class. Since I hadn't planned on attending, my attire was less than suitable. I had on leggings with a short T-shirt that was covered by a long denim jacket fastened up to cover a multitude of sins. Knowing that I couldn't dance in the jacket, I decided to tie it round my waist in the hope that it would cover my wobbly bits as I began to bounce around the room like a fairy elephant.

My petite-to-the-point-of-malnourished American dance teacher was having none of it. 'Take that jacket from round your waist,' she said, crisply enunciating every word to show her disapproval.

'I can't do that,' I said, pleading with her with my eyes to leave me alone.

'Just take it off,' she said impatiently. 'What is your problem?'

'I just want to leave my jacket on,' I said. I could feel

tears springing into my eyes. I was turning red and felt sweat trickling down my face and back.

I weighed about 17 stone 7 pounds at the time, and all the other members of the class were now gazing at me far more intently than they would have done had I been allowed to get on and dance in my camouflage gear.

'Take your jacket off or leave this class,' she persisted. 'Unless you do as you're told, you won't be able to proceed on this course.'

I quickly considered my options, knowing that if I told her the real reason it would be too much to bear and I'd never recover from the humiliation of actually admitting to a room full of teenagers that I was ashamed and embarrassed about my shape. I genuinely believe that I have been spared so many of the cruel and offensive jibes that assail most fat people because I appear not to care, so I don't look vulnerable or easy prey. Showing how I really felt was not an option as it would leave me open to ridicule. Trying to sound cocky and carefree when I felt anything but, I retorted, 'I'll leave.'

I was gutted and walked home feeling extremely distressed. I felt my dance teacher had not only touched my Achille's heel, she had picked it up, squeezed it and then ground it underfoot as if she was stubbing out a cigarette.

I walked home, crying all the way. My mum tried to soothe me as best she could, but however much she wished it, it wasn't in her power to make her unhappy daughter slim.

That was it for me. I wasn't going to go back there to put myself through that kind of humiliation again – I just couldn't face it. So six weeks into my course, I dropped out, and my Saturday job at Evans became full time.

At the time my link back into the acting world was through David Johnson's theatre group. We did a bit of everything, from plays to improvisation. One day, David organised for us to have a session with Michelle Smith, a real casting agent, who came in to do mock auditions for an advert – it had already been cast, so this was just to give us practice at auditioning. On that day I was feeling reasonably confident – I was one of the more experienced members of the group and probably of all of us, the one that was expected to do well. As we waited for our feedback, one of my friends whispered, 'You'll be all right, Mikyla'.

But instead, Michelle went through everyone else, giving comments, but didn't mention me. When she said 'Is that everyone?' I made a point of saying, 'Em, no – you didn't say anything about me.'

'Oh, yes,' she said, looking me up and down. 'Have you heard of Lisa Riley?'

'Yes,' I said, very concerned about what she was going to say. Lisa was at this point doing great work on *Emmerdale*.

'Well, if you're going to look the way you do, you'd better get yourself a personality more like Lisa's.'

Weeks after my fatal dance class, it was another blow to my self-confidence. I wonder, when people make these remarks, if they ever realise how those on the receiving end can remember them for years.

Despite all this though, I persevered. I decided to get myself an agent – albeit not a brilliant one. She was recommended by another girl in the group. The main thing I remember about her was the way she always mispronounced my name. My lovely friend Russell Grant always explains to people how it should be pronounced by saying, 'It's Mikyla the tiler, not Michaela the tailor.'

I was at work one day when my agent called me to ask if I wanted to go for an interview for a small part in *Coronation Street* the following day.

'Can you make it, Kayla? Yes or no?' she said.

Of course I jumped at the chance. The only problem was that it clashed with work.

I begged my boss, Karen, for time off to go for the audition, but she was unsympathetic. 'I don't have anyone else to cover, I'm afraid, Mikyla.'

I was due to finish work at 4 p.m. that day and the audition was an hour later. 'Well, how about just letting me leave fifteen minutes early?' I pleaded. 'I'll never make it otherwise and you know how important it is to me.' I wanted to add, 'This is about my dream. Don't you ever have dreams?' but I thought it would be prudent to keep my mouth shut.

'Well, we'll see, but if the shop's busy, I'm afraid I won't be able to let you go.'

With hindsight I realised I should have pulled a sickie, but my dad had drummed into me from an early age that I should never let people down once I'd committed myself to something.

I spent the next day sweating through every moment, as I tidied rails of clothes, processed credit cards and tried to sound interested in the sartorial dilemmas of women who came into the shop. As I nodded and smiled to the customers, I was fast-forwarding myself to the audition and wondering whether I'd make it in time or not.

At a quarter to four Karen said casually, 'Oh, Mikyla, what are you doing still here?'

I grinned at her and then bolted. There weren't many things that would make me run, probably only an oncoming train or an audition. I ran through the centre of Blackburn faster than I'd ever run before. The Asian boys called out, '*Matee javee*,' a derogatory term for a fat person. I didn't have time to stand and argue with them. I shouted, 'Oh, just piss off,' as I ran, but I think my voice got lost on the wind.

My mum, as ever, was waiting to pick me up and she drove at a possibly illegal speed to get me to the audition on time. I got changed in the car and made it to the Granada studios by the skin of my teeth. My mum screeched to a halt and I sprang out of the car like a cop on *Miami Vice*.

'I'm here for an audition,' I said breathlessly to the woman on reception. I wanted her to be in as much of a rush as I was to direct me to the right place, but she was maddeningly slow.

'Who are you here to see?' she asked.

My mind had gone blank. 'Oh, no, I can't remember the name of the casting director,' I said anxiously.

'What show are you here for?' said the receptionist, rolling her eyes.

'Oh, *Coronation Street*,' I said.

'OK, you want Judi Hayfield, third floor,' she said.

Judi had a reputation as a demi-god in the industry. I was ushered into her room. She was searching through some papers with her back to me and without turning round, said, 'Please sit down. I'll be with you in a minute.'

After a minute or two she came and sat down opposite me and smiled broadly.

'Hello, Mikyla, nice to meet you. We're looking for someone to play a nanny working for Ken Barlow, Bill Roache's character.'

I presumed she would ask me to read something, but instead she just wanted to chat.

'Just tell me what you think makes a good nanny,' she said.

I decided that they wanted a jolly, fat girl for the role and said that I loved children and would just play myself.

She seemed pleased and started talking about filming dates, about how well I'd fit in with the regulars and who would be directing the episode.

Oh, my God, I'm going to get a part in *Corrie*, I thought to myself. The day of anxious sweating at Evans, the sprint to my mum's car and the frantic drive into Manchester were all looking worthwhile.

'I'll get in touch with your agent,' she said. 'You should be hearing from us very soon.'

I got up to say goodbye, and she put her hand over her mouth. I had no idea why but I knew that in a split second everything had gone from perfectly fine to horribly wrong.

'I'm so sorry, Mikyla, I had no idea you were so tall. I'm afraid Sally's only five foot three inches tall and Bill Roache is five foot nine – it just won't work.'

I struggled to understand why it was such a major problem, but now, after years on a soap, I can understand how difficult it makes two shots if the actors are very different heights from each other, especially for a nanny and her two employers.

I shrugged and smiled and pretended it didn't matter. 'Don't worry, that's the way things go.'

'I'm truly sorry, Mikyla. It was really lovely to meet you.'

As I walked out of the room I groaned. Not only was I too fat and too ginger, I was now too tall as well. My initial reaction was to walk out into the street and emit a very loud scream in a bid to empty out my frustrations. But after a few minutes I began to feel much more positive.

Well, at least I was rejected for being too tall rather than because I was too crap or too ugly, or worse still, lacking in personality, as suggested by Ms Smith. I told myself in an attempt to 'therapise'.

By the time I got back to the car, where my mum was waiting for me, I was smiling.

'Well?' she said expectantly.

'I didn't get the part,' I said. 'I was too tall.'

My mum seemed more disappointed than me and saw the fact that I was rejected because I was too tall as a personal affront. I felt more upbeat about the whole experience. I know that I could have thrown myself on my bed and wailed about the fact that a cruel quirk of genetics had snatched a great role away from me, but instead I looked upon the whole experience as a ringing endorsement for my acting ability and good practice at dealing with the inevitable knocks that the tough world of acting would hand out to me. I was still convinced that although I had failed to secure a part this time, my big break was only a matter of time.

10

A Heavy Age

24 stone 7 pounds

I spent five years at Evans and became branch manager, but I knew I needed to move on at some point. I was comfortable there and had done well to get promoted at such a young age. But it wasn't the career I wanted. I was now twenty, and I knew I was never going to have the freedom to chase my dream by going to auditions while stuck in the straitjacket of retail management.

I thought an office job would be slightly more flexible, so with no IT skills and a typing speed of 11 words per minute, I started looking around. But first I had to secure a reference. Who could be more perfect than my old boss from Evans, Karen, who had given me my first job? I put in a long-overdue call and told her my plans.

'You want to work in an office? Are you mad? You were made for retail!' After I explained my reasoning, she shouted to her husband, Tony, 'Will you give Mikyla a job at your office?'

Next thing I knew I had secured a position at TNT in Ramsbottom. I had a desk, a computer and absolutely no clue what I was supposed to be doing.

But I learnt fast. Once again I got promoted and was

awarded 'Employee of the Month'. I started to panic. Yet another career path that wasn't on my original agenda was emerging. 'I'm not a celebrity, get me out of here,' I shouted silently.

As far as food was concerned, this was one of the worst periods in my life. I ate and ate and ate all day. Unlike Evans, where I was at least on my feet all day, here I only moved from my desk to go to the subsidised canteen, a short walk away. Subsidised meant that all our meals were very cheap and almost charged at cost. There was also the dreaded drive home, which was like running a gauntlet, passing one drive-thru, then another, then another . . . It's strange how low-cost, bad food somehow seems less of a sin because you're taking advantage of a bargain. An 'extra-value' this or a '99p' that was just too good to miss, I reasoned.

In so many cases cheap food is bad for us because it's processed and poor quality. It is possible to prepare healthy, nutritional food at a reasonable price, but that doesn't interest the fast-food giants. The adults are seduced by price and the children by toys and other gimmicks, and also the stuff is addictive.

During my TNT days my intake could only be described as obscene. An average day consisted of:

Cereal and toast – at home
Potato cake with lashings of butter – early-morning tea break
Bacon and sausage sandwich – mid-morning tea break
Two white rolls with ham, cheese and coleslaw – lunch
Packet of crisps and a chocolate bar – lunch

Ice cream – afternoon tea break
Double cheese burger and chips – drive-thru on the way
  home
Wholesome home-cooked meal – dinner
500-millilitre tub of Häagen-Dazs – evening TV snack

I look back at that time with sadness and confusion. I had
gone into self-destruct mode without realising it. It
seemed I was on a life-support machine and to keep
me breathing I needed a constant flow of food. I literally
overate as if my life depended on it. The only thing that
put a real smile on my face was stuffing food into my
mouth. I switched off from thinking about what I was
eating. A full mouth and a full stomach were the only
things that made me happy. I became obsessed with pre-
empting feelings of hunger. Those feelings scared me and I
wanted to avoid them at all costs. I had come to the
conclusion that my eating habits and body weight were
unsalvageable and so I might as well just surrender myself
to gorging myself for ever.

There were times when I seemed happy, but those
moments were simply performances that I staged for the
benefit of others. I had retained the desire I had in childhood to please others, but inside I was suffocating.

My twenty-first birthday was fast approaching, as was
my top-scoring weight of 24 stone 7 pounds. For me, it was
more of a case of key to the fridge than key to the door.

Not wanting to have one giant party as most people do, I
decided to have several small affairs over the course of a
couple of weeks. On the actual day itself I opted to go ten-
pin bowling with all my work friends as I remembered

enjoying it so much a few years before. But something had changed – the width of my arse.

This effectively meant I couldn't pull the bowling ball back or launch it in a straight line, as it needed to do a four-mile trip round my bum and hips. Needless to say, I didn't win, as most of my attempts ended in the gutter. I wanted the ground to swallow me up, not because I had lost but because I feared almost everyone there had figured out why I had such difficulty.

In true Mikyla style, I hid my distress well with a blunt, seemingly carefree remark: 'I lost 'cos my arse is so big and I can't throw the bloody ball in a straight line,' I confided, giggling.

My remark was met with a roar of laughter. The others were reassured that I was comfortable with my size so that made it OK.

Next came a weekend in London that my cousin Kim had thoughtfully organised. It involved theatre, shopping and a family dinner. Fortunately this all took place on one day so I could wear the same clothes throughout. At the time I only had one outfit that I felt was acceptable, and trying to find another would have crucified me. It was a pair of brown trousers with a loose-fitting black tunic top that covered my bum.

First stop was Oxford Circus. I always got excited at the prospect of shopping, but never failed to be disappointed. I think my excitement was learnt behaviour from my sister Ella, who loved to shop so much it totally took over her life. She very cleverly balanced an array of credit cards to ensure maximum spending power and minimum interest charged – a talent she passed on to yours truly. I dreamt of being able to walk down the street like Julia Roberts in *Pretty Woman* with bags of clothes, but the similarity ended with the red hair. In reality I was lucky to find even one item that I thought looked good.

And busy Oxford Street for someone my size was hell on earth. It could only just accommodate my body width, without adding a dozen carrier bags which took up yet more precious pavement space. Negotiating busy places is never easy for anybody, but when you're the size of a small house, it is almost impossible. If you attempt it, it's more than likely beads of sweat will roll down your brow as you try to keep up with the other agile pedestrians, who sigh and tut at you, sometimes muttering insults under their breath just loud enough for only you to hear. One person hissed under her breath when she felt I'd invaded her space, 'What is it with fat people?'

However, despite all these trials and tribulations, I was determined to find something acceptable to wear. At size 28, I was now at a point where my shopping options were massively restricted so at least 50 per cent of my wardrobe came from my old stomping ground – Evans. Kim was more than happy for me to take my time. As we wandered in, I starting scouring the racks looking for the new lines we didn't have up North. We methodically worked through each rail to ensure we saw every possible item.

Kim even selected items for 'What do you think of this?' comments. Invariably my answer was 'No', as although the items were nice, they wouldn't flatter me. Eventually she found something I liked so of course she needed to know my size.

'Twenty-eight,' I shouted without hesitation or embarrassment.

Once she had selected the top in my size, she held it up and studied it and then asked casually, 'Mik, do you ever think they will soon run out of sizes to fit you?'

You could have heard a pin drop. Everybody turned to look at her. This is the one place on earth slim people don't pass comment on their fat counterparts. Not EVER.

I swiftly and sharply retorted, 'No, Kim. No I don't, thank you.' She had not meant the remark unkindly, but it cut me to the quick.

I rushed into the fitting room fighting back tears. It wasn't surprising that I didn't make a purchase. My self-esteem had hit the floor with a thud. It's really true that the ones closest to you have the ability to hurt you the most because you least expect them to. If anybody else had asked such a question, I'd have put them firmly in their place, but I knew Kim had no comprehension of what she had said so I couldn't retaliate.

I recovered swiftly and became increasingly excited at the prospect of seeing a matinée of *Saturday Night Fever* at the Palladium. Thanks to Phil and Kim's connections, we had managed to wangle excellent seats at the front of the dress circle. As we climbed the stairs, I could feel my heart racing and I prayed this was the only flight I would be faced with as another could have finished me off. As we started the steep descent to the seats and tried to work out where our seats were, Kim noticed that the seats had full panels to divide them and the space between wasn't very generous.

'Aren't you worried you won't fit in the seat?' she said.

Oh, my God, I thought, what is it with this woman?

Maybe tonight's restaurant overbooked and she's hoping I'll top myself and inadvertently cancel dinner, avoiding any embarrassment on her part.

Again I responded with a simple, 'No, Kim. No I'm not.'

During the first half of the show I comforted myself with a box of Maltesers. In the interval I shot out of my seat to the toilets and rang my mum to rant about Kim's clumsy comments, which resulted in yet more tears.

She tried desperately to reason with me and calm me down. Eventually the bell rang and I was forced to return to my seat, which was admittedly exceedingly snug. So snug in fact that it left an indentation in the side of each upper thigh where my fat had been dragged forward. Looking back, I knew that Kim meant nothing by it and that they were innocent comments – maybe I was over-reacting because I felt so vulnerable.

The show itself was amazing, and I watched the svelte, toned little dancers dart across the stage with ease and grace. Meanwhile there I was, barely able to walk up a flight of stairs or even sit comfortably. Cramming my ample bottom into a theatre seat wasn't the only indignity of being the size I was. I had developed a kind of nappy rash between my thighs as a result of the constant chafing. In the end I had to wear cycle shorts under my clothes to prevent this. And new stretch marks appeared daily, angry red ones that faded to silver.

Later my mum and dad joined us for dinner. My mum had sneaked a cake down from Blackburn with my name iced on it and twenty-one candles. Even my dad behaved himself, although he was probably on pain of death from my mum if he upset me on my big day. But my weight even intruded into my happiness at the meal. When it came to blowing out my birthday candles, I was sitting on a hard, wooden seat. The sides dug into the back of my legs and my arse bulged over either side, making everything very painful.

After my birthday I returned to work with a heavy heart and a deep sense of loneliness that grew the more I pretended I was happy with my appearance. I was now at a stage where all my brother's rants of 'Nobody wants to see a fat person on telly' started to ring true. I decided that the only role I would ever get would be playing a character ridiculed for my size. I had always hoped that I would be considered for the same role as any other female actress but knew that now I was too vast for that to happen. I decided that it would no longer be possible for me to play a normal character simply on the basis of my talent or ability. But I couldn't have been more wrong.

11

'You Can't Start a Diet on a Thursday'

24 stone 7 pounds

The very next day my phone rang. 'Hello, Kayla, I've got an audition lined up for you. It's for a film and they want overweight girls,' said my agent matter-of-factly.

A film! My heart began to race. I'd never auditioned for a movie before. I was absolutely thrilled. It was just the thing I needed to lift me out of the TNT doldrums. I had a gut feeling that this was it. My big break had finally arrived and my days of working in an office were over. Feverishly my brain went into fast-forward mode, wondering who my co-stars might be, whether the film would be a success in the UK or even in the hard-to-crack US market.

My agent sounded distinctly less excited than I was. As ever she didn't sound particularly interested in the progression of my career. The information she had about the film was minimal.

But I scribbled down the details and got straight on the phone to my faithful mum, to enlist her as a chauffeur to the audition in Leeds.

I thought I looked great, but I cringe now thinking about my audition outfit. I was between a size 26 and 28 at the time and wore faux-leather pants and a dazzling orange top with a tie-dye design. I'd put a bright-red rinse on my hair. I looked as if I'd been Tangoed or, worse, as if I was about to burst into flames. I was wearing ankle boots that were too small for my ankles and dug into the fat so that it hung over the sides of the boots, but thankfully it was hidden under my trousers. I was still consuming food at an alarming rate. Whenever I passed a food shop I felt the urge to go in and buy something. I developed strategies to make my enormous consumption less embarrassing, like pretending that I'd come in to buy a very specific item for a friend. I doubt that my performance ever fooled the shop assistants.

I walked into the hotel lobby. It was old and musty with a dark, patterned carpet. I sat on one of the faded sofas and waited. And waited. And waited. I was expecting the film crew to have booked a large room or suite of rooms in which to conduct the auditions, but there was no sign of them, and no sign of any other actors attending the auditions.

Eventually a small woman emerged blinking into the lobby and said in a heavy German accent, 'Mikyla, hello. I am Imogen. You look fabulous, Mikyla. You have so much confidence. I like it already. Now sit down and tell me all about yourself.'

Despite my brash appearance, I instantly went into putdown mode. 'Well, I haven't got much on my CV, just some bits of theatre,' I said.

'No, no, no, I want to hear about *you*,' she breathed, leaning closer and looking at me expectantly, assuming that I would obediently spill a lifetime of intimate secrets into her lap.

I wondered if the whole thing was an elaborate set-up that my agent had gone along with. I expected Jeremy Beadle to leap out at any moment.

'How do your family feel about your weight?' she asked.

'I don't know, we don't really discuss it,' I replied '. . . I've got a brother who's a bit overweight and a sister who's anorexic.'

'Is that because she was too fat to start with?' she asked.

'I don't think so.' I shrugged.

'Tell me all about your brother,' she breathed.

After every comment I made, she gave me a piercing stare as if she was trying to excavate my soul and said, 'How do you feel about that?' or, 'What does your mother say?'

I tried to say everything I thought she wanted me to. I'll say I was locked in a cupboard until I was five if you'll give me a job, I thought to myself. Thankfully I didn't need to resort to fiction.

'I think you'll be perfect for the lead in my film,' she said.

I couldn't believe what I was hearing. I wanted to fling my arms round her neck with gratitude.

'I think we have everything we need. I'll speak to your agent. The next time I meet you will be in London.'

When I emerged from the hotel and found my mum waiting in the car, she was frantic.

'You were in with her for an hour and a half, you know – I thought you'd been kidnapped!'

'Mum, she wants me to be the lead,' I said, so overwhelmed with emotion that my voice wobbled with happy tears.

My mum seemed even more excited than I was. Both of

us drove back to Blackburn in a state of euphoria. But it didn't last. For two months I heard nothing.

I sunk into a deep gloom. I had prayed that this film would be my passport out of TNT, and that if it wasn't going to catapult me into Hollywood stardom, at the very least it would help me to get my name and face known on the British film circuit. I had entirely given up hope when the phone rang once again.

'Keyla, I've had the Imogen woman on the phone again. She wants you to go for an audition in London tomorrow but won't be able to pay your travel expenses. Is that all right, then?'

Of course it was all right. If I had to charter a plane myself, I'd get there. I chose the rather cheaper option of calling on my trusty mum to lend me the money for the train fare. I had to present myself at an address in Finchley Road in the Swiss Cottage area. I'd been told to prepare a Salome dance, but I had no idea what such a thing was.

The building I had to go to was behind heavy iron gates. I pressed a buzzer, spoke into the intercom and the gates swung open. I walked through an ivy-covered arch and started to climb a flight of stairs to Imogen's office. Suddenly I felt very apprehensive. But I had no choice now I'd come all this way. I took a deep breath and got on with it.

'Hello, Mikyla,' she said, shaking my hand vigorously. 'Have you prepared your Salome dance?'

'What do you mean?' I asked.

'It's an emotional tool,' she said, leaving me feeling even more confused. She put on some music and I started swaying in a way that I hoped approximated to a Salome dance, whatever that might be. She stopped the music.

Not surprisingly my rendition wasn't correct. Imogen demonstrated the dance, rubbing her arms up and down her body. Then she said abruptly, 'Right, we have enough of the dancing. How do you feel about nudity?'

That was not a question I had been anticipating, but by now I no longer expected that anything normal would come out of Imogen's mouth. She pulled out a postcard of a pair of breasts with whiskers painted on them.

'In the film the man who plays your boyfriend paints on your boobies and sells postcards of the pictures. You will need to get your boobies out.'

I had been momentarily struck dumb, but I soon found my voice again: 'There is no way I'm going to do that,' I said. 'No way on this earth.'

She looked terribly disappointed. 'In that case I can't give you the lead role in the film,' she said. 'This is very saddening for me.' Then she seemed to overcome her disappointment. 'Well, there are other roles you could play. Do you think you could do sumo wrestling?'

This was another surprise. 'I could have a go,' I said, not wanting to give another negative response. It wasn't quite what I had envisaged my first role in a bona fide film to be, but I clung on to the hope that this could be my big break.

So, with me having accepted a lesser role, in October 1998 we began the sumo training for *Secret Society*. The film was a romantic comedy, with Lee Ross and Charlotte Brittain playing the lead roles, and Annette Badland in a character role. It plots the story of Daisy, an overweight girl who gets a job in her local factory. She soon realises that there are a number of fat women there who appear to get preferential treatment, including specially prepared lunches of gargantuan proportions. After a number of initiation tests Daisy is invited to join their secret society . . . a secret society of sumo wrestlers.

All the other actresses apart from me had equity cards and they all came from London or other parts of the South. I was the only Northerner, and without an equity card I felt like the underdog, the country bumpkin of the film. But I enjoyed the challenge of the sumo wrestling and got along very well with our trainer, Sid. Before starting training, I had assumed that I'd have to practise a handful of moves a few times and that 100 per cent precision would not be expected or required. That comfortable assumption was soon shattered and the punishing training schedule we were expected to stick to was revealed. Sumo wrestling is an official martial art, and I discovered there's a lot more to it than there looks. After the first training session I felt so stiff I could barely put one foot in front of the other. The training lasted eight weeks and we had three sessions a week.

'I can't go on, Sid,' I groaned over and over again, as he demanded more and more from me and the other girls.

'Yes, you can,' he replied placidly, impervious to emotional blackmail of any description. 'If you're going to do this, it's very important to do it properly.'

He was right, and by the end of the eight-week training period I had become, if not an accomplished sumo wrestler, certainly a passable one. The complexities of wrapping the long linen sash nappy-style round me no longer baffled me. I could assemble this cloth contraption almost as quickly as I could tie my shoelaces.

Once I'd got the hang of the training I loved the moves. I was really looking forward to starting filming and was sure the film would be a great success. Then, out of the blue, my dreams were shattered. I got a phone call one morning to say the whole thing had been called off. I didn't fully take in the news at first and thought it was just the coming week's training session that had been cancelled. But it was the entire film. Apparently £2 million had already been spent even though not a single frame had been shot. I went into shock. I couldn't believe that something so official and costing so much money could suddenly collapse.

I was devastated that a role I had worked so hard for and sweated over so profusely had been cruelly snatched away from me.

As usual, though, I tried to salvage a bleak situation. Throughout the training period I had kept remembering my pledge to myself that as soon as the film was wrapped up I was going to start dieting in earnest. That moment had arrived sooner than I'd expected.

The rest of the cast were as miserable about the cancellation of the film as I was, and we all went out and got blindingly drunk to drown our sorrows. Strangely, this was the closest I ever felt to the rest of the cast. We seemed to do some bonding that day. Adversity does bind people together, and for the first time I felt equal to the other women. I woke up the next morning horribly hungover but still resolute about losing weight. I staggered downstairs, to Kim and Phil, with whom I was staying in Harrow.

'You look a real sight,' Kim said to me. 'I'll make you a big breakfast – cereal, toast and jam with tea and two sugars. That should banish your hangover and soak up some of that alcohol.'

I shook my head firmly. 'No. I'm going to have a piece of dry toast and a banana. I've decided that today I'm going to start my diet. I promised myself that I would start to diet properly as soon as the film was over. Today's the day and I need to start right now.'

She looked at me in disbelief. 'You can't start a diet on a Thursday,' she tutted. 'No one starts a diet on a Thursday. Why not wait until next week and start then?'

'No, I'm going to start now,' I said.

Losing weight is like any other life change. Fads and miracle cures will never work alone, but if there is sincere and determined motivation, change will come. For a long time I had been lacking that motivation. I had been on diets in the past that never worked because I missed calorie-laden food too much. I knew at that hungover moment that either I could carry on eating and gain another 5 stone and that eventually I would pop or I could take myself in hand, lose 5 stone and get my body back to a more manageable size.

Despite her initial reaction, Kim was extremely supportive as soon as she and Phil realised that I was serious and that this was a turning point. I was experiencing a kind of epiphany. They pulled out all the stops, giving me their expensive exercise bike, which was loaded into the boot of my Escort. They gave me advice about vitamin supplements and gave me my new bible – Oprah Winfrey's book *Make the Connection*. For the first time in my life that's exactly what I did. I made the connection between my body, my brain and what I tipped into my mouth on a daily basis.

I was phenomenally disciplined, although at times I

wanted certain foods so badly that I cried. I could have committed murder for a chip buttie or a tub of Häagen-Dazs, but I resisted. I lived on grilled chicken, ham, low-fat coleslaw, stir-fried vegetables and jacket potatoes. If I ate fattening things, I ate them in minute quantities and I tipped copious amounts of salt, pepper and mustard on to any leftovers in case I was tempted to eat them. I religiously spent twenty minutes every morning on Kim and Phil's exercise bike. For the first time in my life I dipped into the psyche of my sister Sam and could understand her anorexia. I had no control over the collapse of the film, no control over being single and no control over the way my dad spoke to me because I was living under his roof and couldn't afford to move out. Food was the only thing I still had some power over, and by refraining from stuffing myself I felt that I had regained a modicum of self-respect.

My sister Ella ran a craft shop, and when the film collapsed she offered me a job working with her. Having given up my job and told people that I was appearing in a film, it was humiliating to end up working for my sister, although I know that I was lucky to have a job at all.

Ella was wonderful. She sat and cried for me, 'You were very brave and tried to follow your dreams. It's not fair what happened to you. I just wish I could fix things for you. I'm so cross about all of this. You really don't deserve it.'

I ended up comforting her. 'Don't worry, Ella. I'll be fine,' I said. 'These things happen for a reason.'

Ella had been on holiday to St Lucia several times and on one of the trips had met a man called Precious. None of us had any idea about the relationship until she called me and asked me to pick her up from the airport on her return from one of her trips. 'I'm bringing something back with me,' she said cagily.

I thought that maybe she'd bought a bulky item of furniture or excessive duty-free and went to the airport to meet her with Rosco. She approached us beaming. Standing behind her was a man she introduced as Precious. She explained she'd met him in St Lucia.

Rosco clapped his hand over his mouth at the sight of Ella with a black man in tow. 'Oh, my God, Grandad Glenn is going to flip,' he said.

Rosco was right. Recently when my mum and I were chatting idly about the kind of man I'd like to marry, I said casually to her, 'You never know – I might end up marrying a black man.'

My dad's face turned thunderous. 'Fucking serious. I'd rather you turned out to be a lesbian than marry a nigger,' he said.

My dad wasn't impressed with Ella's choice of man, in fact he was furious. But she was a grown woman and not his daughter, so there wasn't much he could do. Precious spent the next few years travelling between St Lucia and Blackburn, and he and Ella married and had two children together, Cameron and Preshella, who are my little angels.

My relationship with Ella continued to be a close one after Precious's arrival, and as always she sweetly encouraged me to achieve whatever I wanted.

And I did. By May 1999, six months after the film was cancelled, I had lost 5 stone. I was overjoyed that I was disciplined enough to eat sensibly after years of piling more and more rubbish into my mouth. My dad had unkindly called me the 'human waste-disposal unit', but he wasn't wrong.

I was still overweight but so many of the flabby lumps and bumps had gone. I looked more streamlined in my clothes, and what mattered more to me than the way I looked was the fact that I did have some willpower and I could be mistress of my own BMI destiny. I was thrilled and vowed to continue with my reduced eating plan. I was determined that I would never again allow my weight to creep up to 24 and a half stone. I loved feeling more energetic and less breathless, I loved wearing clothes that felt comfortably loose instead of cutting harshly into my waist and arms, and I loved being able to say to myself and others that I had taken control of my destiny. A particular triumph was being able to weigh myself on ordinary bathroom scales. Most scales only go up to 20 stone, so for the first few months of my diet, to chart my weight loss, I had to suffer the humiliation of standing on the big scales in Boots that you put 10 pence into. My family encouraged me, and my cousin Kim was particularly supportive, calling me every week to see how I was getting on and congratulating me warmly each time a few more pounds rolled off my bones.

Before I embarked on my diet, I felt that I had slid off the edge of the cliff and was freefalling into the sea. The weight loss made me feel as if somehow I had made a superhuman effort to clamber back on to the edge of the cliff. I was still staring into the abyss, but I was no longer tumbling headlong into it. My mum and Ella were very proud of me, although my dad said very little about it all.

I had more or less resigned myself to the cancellation of

the film and was feeling reasonably contented about continuing to lose weight and having a job that paid me enough money to get by. After a couple of months I got a job working for an underwear shop. My agent called me and told me I had an audition for a small part in the BBC2 show *Cops*. I hated the job at the shop and knew I wouldn't be given time off to go to the audition. I tried to fit the audition in during my lunch hour, hoping it would be quick. In fact it lasted all afternoon and I simply never went back to my job – something I'd never done before or since. I got the part in *Cops*, and although it was small, I was praised for my portrayal at the screening. Next I got a job at a card chain, which I also loathed. I broke my foot while working there, but there was no sympathy or flexibility from my bosses.

Then, out of the blue, I got a phone call. The film was back on. Did I want to get involved again? A million thoughts went through my mind. I was terrified of agreeing to get involved only to find that once again the project fell apart before the cameras started rolling. But I also knew that if I turned down the opportunity and the film ended up being a hit at the box office, I'd never forgive myself. And even if it wasn't a runaway success, I'd still have it on my CV.

'OK, then,' I said, taking a deep breath. 'I'll give it another go. When do I start?'

We began work again in June 1999. With most of the things I've done in my life, either school, office work or acting, I've made friends. But this film was an exception. There was no sense of a happy reunion when I saw the cast members again. Nobody congratulated me on my weight loss. I wondered if it was not the done thing in fat circles to make overt references to weight loss – as if shedding pounds was somehow letting the fat side down. In theory, being surrounded by fat women should have made me feel at ease – they ranged from a size 18 to a size 30 – but for some reason I felt very uneasy in the company of this group of women. They were prepared to chat in general terms about their lives and the irritating on-off nature of the film, but we never discussed anything personal at all.

One person who did notice my weight loss, though, and was extremely unhappy was Imogen. She took a long, hard look at me when I arrived back on set and said sternly, 'Hmm, you've lost weight. No more!'

It was a surreal moment, the first time in my life that I'd been instructed not to lose weight. The filming took place on the edge of Doncaster and we stayed at the Moat House Hotel nearby. I think that anyone who saw the group of us together assumed that we were part of a delegation for a WeightWatchers convention – and not a very successful one at that.

All the sumo girls were caked in thick white make-up. This deathly pale gunge was much harder to remove from a fat body than a thin one because it lodged in all the crevices where rolls of fat pooled. When we swam in the hotel pool to relax after shooting, we were like a school of graceful whales bobbing up and down and the white make-up clogged up the pool filters.

We filmed some of the wrestling scenes in an old, disused warehouse, and one day we had a bunch of unwelcome spectators peering through the windows at us. They were guests on the way to a wedding party, and I heard one of them shout in a broad Doncaster accent, ''Ere, there are ten fat birds painted in white paint, wearing nappy things with their arses out.' So much for the glamorous life of a film star. Talk about 'Beam me up, Scotty'. Suddenly the thought of thousands of people watching us at the cinema made me feel quite ill.

There were some scenes in a Turkish baths, but we were all adamant that we wouldn't do full nudity. Most of us were prepared to allow the towel to slip a little and reveal some flesh on camera, but nobody was prepared to strip off completely – although Imogen would have been delighted if we'd agreed to that.

'Oh, you all look beautiful,' she exclaimed, as we sat with towels draped over us, desperately trying to make them cover as much flesh as possible. Imogen started to move the towels, ostensibly to make our poses look more 'arty', although in fact she was sneakily trying to get more flesh exposed. She was bunching up one girl's towel more and more. Claire was northern Irish and didn't mince her words.

'I'm not having any muff showing and that's final,' said Claire, clamping the towel firmly over her genitals.

'Vot is "muff"?' said Imogen perplexedly. We all howled with laughter.

All in all, the shoot was grim. Imogen had engaged a firm of East German caterers and we were expected to eat goulash every single day.

When we finished filming, the wrap party was rather flat. It was the only time in my life where I'd had a job and made no friends. I knew that I should be feeling overjoyed to have appeared in my first film, but the strangeness of making the film and the lack of bonding amongst the other actors made the whole experience quite miserable. I felt more at home working in Ella's craft shop than on this particular film set. And so ended my first venture on to the silver screen.

12
Meeting Chloe

19 stone 10 pounds

The film was over, and alas, my phone stayed silent. I had to find something that paid the bills. I got a job in Hampson's Bakery, which was a world away from the very peculiar film set I'd spent months on. I found myself serving meat pies and egg-custard tarts to the people of Blackburn. But rather than sinking into gloom at the absence of further acting offers, I enjoyed my days there.

Secret Society was never distributed in the UK, and so I waited, not unhappily, for my big break in acting. I had assumed that because I had done a film, work would fall at my feet, but my phone remained depressingly quiet. It was my friend from school Sonia who got me the job at Hampson's. Her mum was a manager there. Of course a shop filled with pies and cakes and sandwiches was my idea of heaven, but miraculously I remained focused on my diet. We baked pies throughout the day, and the policy of the shop was to have a few of the bestsellers available right up until closing time. Any left then had to be thrown away. I devised certain rules for myself. A couple of times a week I ate the filling and top of a meat and potato pie but would throw away the pastry case. I had a particular weakness for

Bavarian slices – a combination of biscuit pastry, gooey cream, vanilla and icing – but again I managed to ration them so that I kept off most of the weight I'd lost.

From the moment I had decided that I wanted to pursue a career as an actress, I was determined that it wouldn't stop me from living a normal life. I had seen people who were obsessed with the idea of fame and fortune, going to three or four auditions every week and constantly getting knocked back. I knew that that wasn't for me. I would make a life no matter what.

While I worked at Hampson's, I was a size 22. Thankfully they made uniforms big enough to fit me – a yukky creamy-beige uniform, teamed with a maroon apron and a white hat. When I was a little girl and attended the Brownies, my Snowy Owl had to come round to measure me up, then went away to make a uniform for me – I was too big for the off-the-peg ones. I'm guessing she got a special badge for doing that for me. I was determined that the same thing wouldn't happen at Hampson's and that I would not go beyond a size 22.

In between when the film was cancelled and the date we all wrapped, I had gone from 24 stone 7 pounds to 19 stone 10 pounds, despite being surrounded by fattening foods. My agent called me one day while I was tipping hot steak pies with glistening crusts and splodges of fragrant gravy oozing over the sides on to a metal tray.

'Hello, Kayla,' she said. 'Can you make an audition in Liverpool in a couple of hours' time?'

'Yes, yes, of course I can,' I said excitedly. If I was being sent to Liverpool, I thought it was probably for *Brookside*. I looked around at the familiar shelves of the bakery, and even though I was happy, my adrenaline kicked in and I just couldn't wait to get back into audition mode. I knew I could act and I was dying to show a casting director exactly what I could do.

I called my mum breathlessly and asked her if she could drop everything and drive me to Liverpool. Being the devoted mum that she is, she agreed and off we went.

'Just cover for me,' I said to the other staff, as I disappeared out of the door, flushed with anticipation. We stopped off at the hairdresser's, who obligingly blow-dried some life back into my flattened hair. Then I slapped some make-up on in the car.

I arrived and tried to sound cool and confident when I announced myself to the receptionist.

'Hello, I'm Mikyla Dodd, I've come for the audition.'

The receptionist handed me a script with the word '*Hollyoaks*' on the top.

'*Hollyoaks?*' I said. 'I thought I was auditioning for *Brookside.*'

'The part you're reading for is a girl of about seventeen,' said the receptionist a little vaguely.

'Could you tell me where the toilets are?' I said, panicked. I knew that if I was to play a seventeen-year-old I needed to wipe off every trace of make-up pronto – I was twenty-two.

There was some horrible green soap and some coarse paper towels in the toilets. I scrubbed hard at my face with both and got every last trace of make-up off.

Dorothy Andrew was the casting director. I was surprised she didn't seem to recognise me from our recent theatre group showcases.

'Hello, I'm Dorothy Andrew,' she said stiffly.

Then the producer, Jo Hallows, introduced herself. She was absolutely delightful – warm, friendly and generous. She explained a bit about the characters in the scene and said that Dorothy would be reading the scene with me.

'You're reading for the part of Chloe,' she said. 'She's a large girl, but she's beautiful, savvy and very direct, OK?'

I nodded eagerly.

'She's the kind of girl who, if someone said, "Oy, fat girl," to her, she'd retort, "Oy, ugly bloke." She's strong and bright.'

I put my heart and soul into the reading. Dorothy, reading with me, had the script held up close to her face. As a result I had no facial expressions or eye contact from her to help me along. Exasperated, I pulled her script down a little, revealing her face.

'Oh, there you are,' I said chirpily. 'Is it all right for me to see your face?'

'All right, then,' said Dorothy.

Jo asked me to read more and more. She was enthused and encouraging. She asked my age.

I half whispered, 'Twenty-two,' which I knew was rather old to play a seventeen-year-old.

Then she asked what my last job had been.

'I played a sumo wrestler in a film. I had to wear a big nappy thing.' I grinned. Jo laughed too. 'But right now I work in a pie shop,' I added. 'Please give me a job!'

'I'll be in touch soon,' Jo said.

I jumped into the car, where my mum was waiting.

'I think it went well,' I said cautiously, as we drove back to Blackburn.

Aged just three in one of my Norma Desmond moods

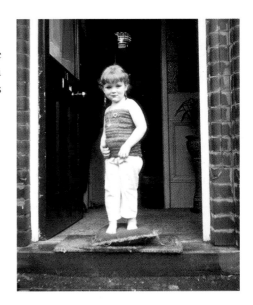

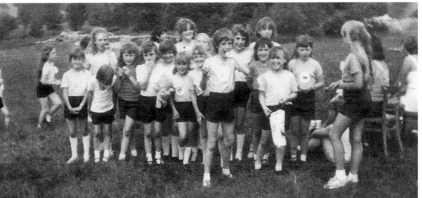

In Brownies - I was seven, five foot four and 7 stone

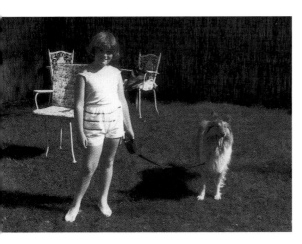

In Germany with my only playmate

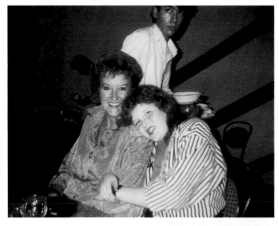

Aged eight with my mum in a restaurant full of adults, as usual

Another restaurant . . .

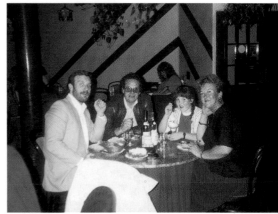

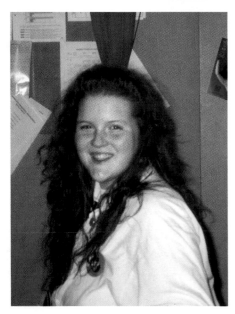

Aged fourteen, 14 stone. This was around the time of the termination. I cut off my hair after Kal and I finally broke up.

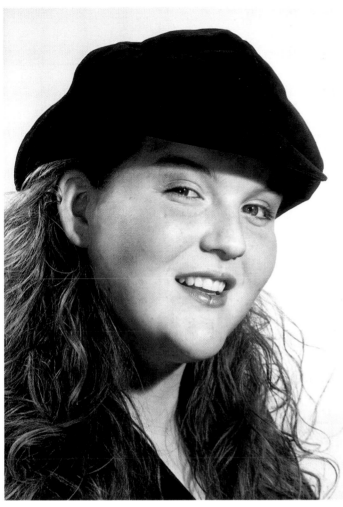

My first acting 10x8, wearing
my Eponine hat like the girl
in *Les Miserables* - we all had
to have these.

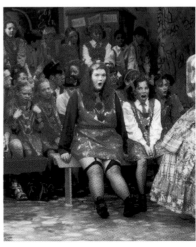

Doing panto, aged fifteen,
and 16 1/2 stone

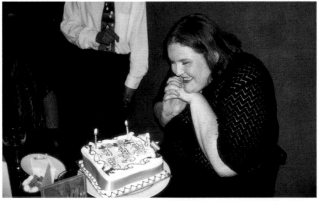

My twenty-first birthday. It was a case of the keys to the fridge rather than the door.

With my sister Ella, feeding our shopping addiction at the Trafford Centre, Manchester, though it's hard to find clothes when you're this size – I was at my biggest, a size 26-28.

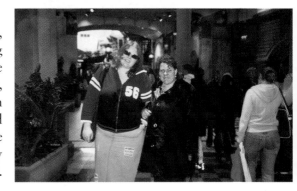

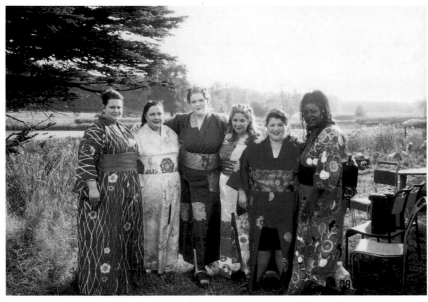

On the set of *Secret Society* having lost some weight – believe it or not, I was bigger when we first started the film.

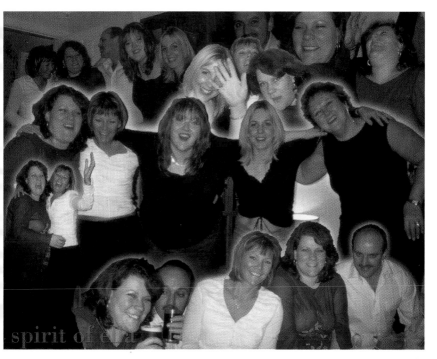

Spirit of Ella – we made this family collage after Ella passed away.

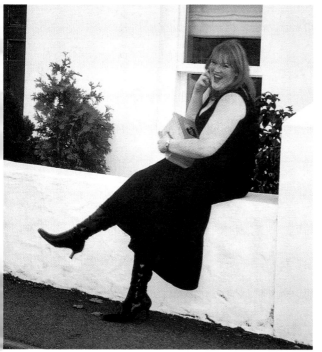

In Guernsey with Ella – I left the wake with her ashes. Our last picture together.

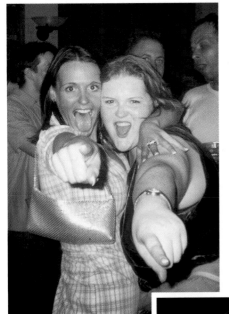

With Sarah (Suranne) Jones at my second soap awards, which was her first - feeling great with my old pal beside me.

With Gary Lucy, my best mate, just before beginning a big diet - I weighed 21½ stone.

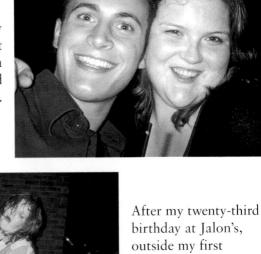

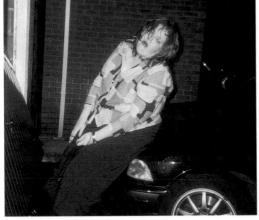

After my twenty-third birthday at Jalon's, outside my first house. I was due to get up at 7.30 that morning - in my hand is my phone, which was my alarm.

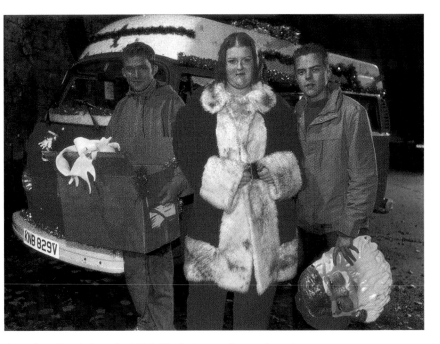

Another 'Let's laugh AT Mikyla' storyline - dressing up as Mother Christmas.

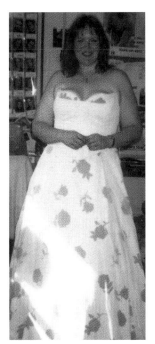

In Chloe's wedding dress, feeling like a princess at 17 1/2 stone. I didn't think there would be a wedding dress my size, but we found one.

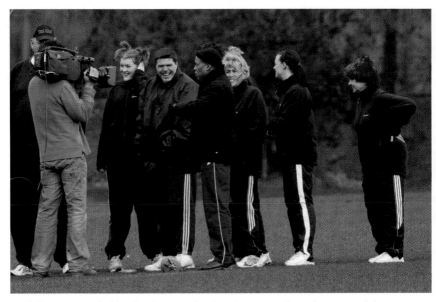

Celebrity Fit Club, which was the final step and took me to fifteen stone - from my heaviest of twenty-four stone, it's been an incredible journey.

Doing a naked photo shoot for a magazine. This would have been my biggest nightmare two years ago - but I loved it!

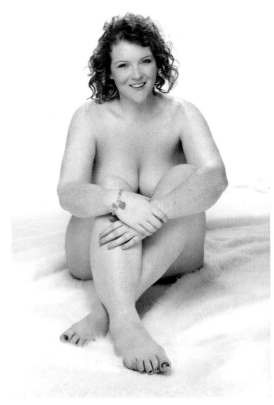

By the time we got home there was a message on the answerphone from my agent.

'Hello, Kayla. You've got the job. Filming starts in three weeks and you've got three episodes.'

My mum and I whooped in unison at the news. I had been so close to giving up hope, but the lovely Jo Hallows had thrown me a lifeline. I trembled with excitement. I had been waiting for this moment for years. *Hollyoaks* was watched by 4 million people, and I prayed that during my three-week run someone would watch my performance, like what they saw and offer me a lead role in a top drama – well, I've always had a fertile imagination!

The first thing I did when I heard the news was run down to Hampson's to tell them I was leaving.

'Don't you think that's a bit risky?' said a couple of the staff. 'Giving up your day job for some temporary acting job.'

I shook my head and smiled. They didn't understand that the bakery job was my temporary job waiting for my real job in acting to begin. At last, it seemed, it had.

I worked out a three-week period of notice at Hampson's. To everyone's amazement, I didn't slacken off or suddenly consider myself to be above unloading steaming pies from the oven. I worked diligently and perhaps even harder than I had before. I was very grateful to have got the job in Hampson's when there was nothing else on the horizon for me, and I didn't want to spit in the company's face now.

Having sold my Escort to cut my financial outgoings, I was without transport so I bought a £300 Fiesta to drive myself between Blackburn and Liverpool every day. At one point my excitement wore off. I was buying myself a rubbish car to go and do a few episodes as a one-off character who would easily be forgotten. Then I brightened and fixed again on all the doors the role of Chloe, *Hollyoaks*'s first fat girl, might open for me.

I arrived at the studios but no one had any record of my name. Being an official non-person was hardly an auspicious start. Finally someone found a record of me somewhere, and I was directed towards make-up and wardrobe. In my first scene Chloe had been set up on a blind date with one of the male characters. I had brought along some black, sparkly outfits that I felt reasonably confident in and thought would be appropriate for a scene in a nightclub.

When I arrived at the wardrobe department and announced myself, a slim blonde woman gestured towards a rail. That's right – even the wardrobe girl was a slim blonde. I wondered if it was a prerequisite to get through the gates, or whether this was some kind of genetic mutation that occurred spontaneously to female cast members once they got on the *Hollyoaks* set. I found out later that although the casting directors did hire some young brunette women, once they joined the cast they started altering their hair colour with subtle highlights at first, gradually getting blonder and blonder. I vowed to protect my ginger tresses.

'That's your outfit for the club scene hanging up there,' said the wardrobe woman. I gazed in horror at what had been picked out for me – a sequinned pink Lycra miniskirt and a little black top with fringing on it. I could see even before I tried it on that the top would be too short for me and would allow my belly to hang over the top.

'I can't wear that,' I gasped. 'I'll look too awful!'

But the wardrobe woman didn't seem to care.

'Surely this can't be right for my costume,' I pleaded. 'I've brought some clothes with me that I think will be much more suitable.'

'I haven't got time for that,' said the wardrobe woman crossly. 'I've been given specific instructions about what you have to wear and that's that.'

She flounced out of the room, and as she went I felt as if she took every ounce of my energy with her, leaving me in a metaphorical dejected heap on the floor.

Jo had described the character to me as a lovable, cool girl, not a laughing stock. I couldn't see how this horrendous outfit, which wouldn't look too good on someone who was a size 12, let alone a woman of 19 stone, fitted the bill.

I fled to the toilets and wept. After a few minutes of sobbing, however, I couldn't see what choice I had other than to put on this hideous combo and allow people to poke fun at me. I cringed as I pulled the Lycra miniskirt over my chunky legs and ginormous bum, and grimaced as the top revealed an expanse of white, floppy flesh round my middle.

Then I washed my face in the hope that I wouldn't look as if I'd been crying and found my way to make-up. A lovely Scottish woman called Marie was there to greet me. She couldn't have been more of a contrast to the woman in wardrobe.

'Hello, Mikyla, pop yourself down there and we'll get you through make-up. Is there any particular sort of look you like?'

As she dabbed and smoothed the contents of different pots and tubes on to my skin, I started to feel better. Just being in Marie's company was soothing. She put some shimmery make-up on my cheeks and I was pleased with the way she transformed my face. Every so often she glanced down at my huge, milky-white, purple-veined thighs, which poked out of my long coat. She said nothing, but I could see that she was thinking, What on earth have they done to this poor girl?

I even longed to be wearing the fishnet tights and leotard that I'd been forced into wearing at Oldham Theatre Workshop. Anything but this.

Wardrobe had assigned me a flimsy pair of open-toed shoes with slender heels. My fat feet hung over the edges, and I was sure that if I leant backwards on the shoes, my weight would quite simply splinter them. I forced myself to lean forwards, putting my weight on the balls of my feet in a bid to avoid that devastating scenario from coming to pass.

For the first scene, which took place in a nightclub, they'd booked space in a downstairs bar of a Liverpool club called the Life Bar. Three male members of the cast, James Redmond, Matt Littler and Darren Jeffries, and I were transported there in a minibus. With my coat clutched round my exposed legs, I was wary of making a fool of myself and kept fairly quiet. The male actors were all deep in conversation about *Star Wars* and didn't pay much attention to me. I was relieved, because I was preoccupied with my disastrous outfit and didn't really feel like making small talk. Because I was so anguished about my clothes, I didn't have time to have more generalised first-day nerves.

The horror of the Lycra miniskirt and skimpy top eclipsed all other thought. I had of course watched *Hollyoaks* before I went for my audition and knew that it was populated by lots of young, blonde women with impossibly slender bodies, but I didn't feel intimidated by the prospect of standing alongside these flimsy creatures.

From the day I embarked on my acting career, I knew that I didn't look like most other actresses and that there were two ways I could respond to this difference – either I could constantly compare myself with others and feel inadequate and defeated or I could look upon every acting job as a great experience and an opportunity to learn as much as I could. I chose the latter, and somehow this residual optimism carried me through the minibus journey in my ghastly get-up.

At one point I even felt bold enough to say to Matt Littler, who plays Max, then a relatively new character on the show, who was Chloe's blind date, 'Do you want to run the scene now?'

He shook his head. 'Not really, we can do it on set.'

I shuddered with embarrassment, though I found out later that the cast often did run through scenes before they got on set.

We arrived at the club and I was thrilled to see that lots of police officers were waiting to greet us. The club was cordoned off with cones.

Wow, I thought, all this for us. My excitement faded, however, when I glimpsed my reflection in a plate-glass office window. I prayed that I was in a dream sequence like in *Ally McBeal* and that in a few moments I'd wake up and find that all was right with my world. We were directed down a spiral staircase to the basement bar. I was convinced I was going to go flying out of my ridiculous shoes. Balancing on the balls of your feet on a narrow spiral staircase when you weigh over 19 stone isn't the easiest or safest thing in the world to do.

Somehow I made it in one piece and Jo was waiting in the basement to greet me.

'Hi, Mikyla,' she said warmly. Then she looked at me. 'Oh, my God, what on earth are you wearing?' she gasped.

'This is what they gave me in wardrobe,' I whimpered.

'Go in there, go in there,' she said firmly, ushering me into the girls' toilets. 'I'll deal with this.' She got on the phone with the wardrobe department and hit the roof. I could hear her say, 'What on earth were you thinking? Mikyla's character is supposed to be dressed in something young and cool and fashionable. This is not what I asked for. Find something better than that for her to wear.'

She asked me what shops I bought my clothes from and dispatched a couple of wardrobe staff to them to find me something more flattering. Jo was wonderful.

'Don't worry, you're not here to be laughed at. We won't do anything until you and I are both happy, OK? I hope this hasn't ruined what should be a really exciting day for you.'

The wardrobe staff returned with some black knee-high boots from Evans, a knee-length black skirt with big red roses on it and a little pink top with a square neck. I put the clothes on and instantly felt better. My hair was back-combed with beautiful little butterfly clips put into it. The reality is that I was never going to look like the rest of the cast: I wasn't blonde, I certainly wasn't slim, and I'd never signed with a modelling agency, unlike so many of the other girls. My legs would never be tanned or dimple-free, and my boobs didn't sit perfectly in front of me like two firm, round melons, rather they hung down like two fat aubergines. But I was happy that at last I looked presentable.

My first scene was dancing in the club. The music was added later, and I worried that I wasn't dancing in time with whatever the eventual beat would be.

'For God's sake, smile and try to look as if you're enjoying yourself,' shouted Jo.

In the scene, Matt Littler appears, full of optimism that he'd been lined up with a gorgeous blind date. Then he sees Chloe and groans, 'Oh, no.' He peers at her through the gloom. 'You've got to be joking. I'm not going on a date with Chloe Bruce the Moose.'

Chloe makes desperate attempts to talk about the things she thinks he wants to talk about, then she tries to make him laugh. In the end she says, 'Well, we're both here now, so why don't we try to enjoy ourselves? All I've done is try to be nice to you. It's not that bad being with me, is it?'

Then he says, 'You're right, I've been a dickhead,' and they get along much better after that.

Next they go back to his place with his mate OB, and when OB insults Chloe, Matt stands up for her and asks him to leave. Then they kiss. I felt that things had gone pretty well up until that point but now I panicked. He was only seventeen and I was twenty-two. I felt like a child-snatcher. And my kissing experience wasn't exactly encyclopaedic. Our lines called for bravado, with both of us falsely boasting that we'd kissed loads of people. I hoped that propping my lips up against his would be sufficient for Jo. The prospect of getting tongues involved filled me with dread. I had only ever kissed a couple of boys, probably because when everybody else was changing boyfriends as often as their clothes, I was wrapped up in Kal. I panicked and thought that maybe he wouldn't kiss the way people from Blackburn kissed.

The snogging scene was going to be filmed in one of the *Hollyoaks* houses, which backed on to the *Brookside* houses. At the time *Hollyoaks* was still the only soap filmed in real houses. It meant that filming could get very cramped, but there was much more scope to get different angles and interesting shots, creating a more real feel to the show. I drove myself to Brookside Close in my Fiesta as it was a weekend night shoot so there was nobody available to pick me up from the main studio. It was so difficult to find, and when I finally arrived there, the security guard at the gate again had no clue who I was. Eventually I was waved through and found my way to make-up, where the lovely Marie was waiting for me once again.

Terri Dwyer had just finished her scene and was wiping her make-up off. She was chatting on her phone, and when she had finished her call, she turned round and said, 'Oh, hi, babe – you've got your kissing scene coming up, haven't you?'

I nodded.

'I was absolutely horrified to hear them call you a moose, and saying all those dreadful things about you,' she added. 'Doesn't it bother you?' Before I could answer, she went on, 'But I suppose that kind of thing is like water off a duck's back to you now.'

Terri is one of my best friends now and I know she intended no malice. Years later I still tease her about this.

At the time, though, I was extremely taken aback and desperately wanted to challenge her. Instead I looked in the mirror at Marie, who mouthed, 'Cheeky cow.'

It's sometimes the case that people don't intend to be cruel or put you down but the words just come out that way. I wonder if people later play the conversation back in their mind and realise their faux pas but are unable to apologise as the apology itself could draw the insulted person's attention to something they had originally missed.

With hindsight I'm glad I didn't challenge Terri, because an unnecessary and bitter exchange could have made it awkward to connect later and I may never have gained such a wonderful friend. Terri of all people appreciates how difficult it is to maintain a slender figure. She is careful with food and works extremely hard at the gym. When I lived with her, this baffled and amused me, but as my attitude to exercise has changed to become an essential part of my daily life, I look at her as an inspiration.

After hair and make-up, continuity was matched up with the previous scene I'd filmed and I had to sit around for another two hours. Then it was time to film again.

First, we did a read-through, followed by a block-through, in which we were given the positions where we were expected to stand or sit, then a rehearsal. Next, the scene was lit, then we did another rehearsal and finally filming. I felt surprisingly calm.

Jo's instructions were for us to 'snog' each other. Once again I agonised about whether the open-lipped or closed-lip option was expected. A few minutes later, after Max and I had daintily touched lips, it became abundantly clear: 'I haven't got time for this,' yelled Jo. 'Get your mouths open, for Pete's sake, and snog. I'm sure you both know how.'

'Do we have to?' said Matt quietly to me.

'Let's just save ourselves embarrassment and get on with it,' I said.

He placed his hand at the back of my head and we snogged beautifully. Jo was satisfied.

Post-snogging, the conversation jumps to them asking each other whether or not they are both virgins. Coyly they admit that they are and agree to relieve themselves of this burden and get down and dirty. We climb under his Action Man duvet and begin fumbling. I had been given a black bra with red roses on and matching knickers by the wardrobe department. Jo assured me that neither my knickers nor the expanse of flesh that separated my bra from my knickers would be shown. I weighed just over 19 stone when I started at *Hollyoaks* and I certainly didn't want my naked body to go on television. Just as the cameras started to roll, the director of photography, who's in charge of lighting, shouted, 'Cut!' Rushing on set, he pulled the duvet up over the top of my fat white arm, the one closest to the camera. He whispered, 'It doesn't look very nice.' Hurtful as that comment was, I was also grateful that he spared me a little on-screen dignity.

Matt was wearing his boxer shorts and as he fumbled Chloe had to say, 'It's not in yet,' followed by a slightly disappointed: 'Is that it?'

In the next scene she's putting her clothes back on.

'Can I see you again?' he asks.

'No, I'm busy,' she jokes.

So ended my first episode on *Hollyoaks*. I was pleased

with the way everything had gone and felt surprisingly relaxed on set.

Jo was also pleased. She approached me at the end of the second day of filming and said, 'I don't know what I'm going to do with you, but would you like to stay beyond the three episodes we've lined up for you?'

'Yes, I really would,' I said to her.

I had no idea then that those three episodes were to turn into nearly five years. The producers kept adding me into scenes, but in my first year on the show my survival was rather hand to mouth. They would ask me if I was available for the next four weeks. Of course I always said that I was, but asking whether I was available and giving me lines were two very different things. I wasn't being paid a retainer, so some weeks when I had no role I earned absolutely nothing, but I couldn't take on any other work because I'd agreed to make myself available to them. That's the downside of life on a soap when you're part of the show but don't have a starring role. I kept reminding myself that Chloe was never intended to be an established character and that I should hang on for dear life and give my all to whatever lines they did give me. By the fourth episode it became apparent that Darren Jeffries, who plays OB, and I had great comic chemistry. We began rehearsing funny scenes and gags together.

Then Matt called me and said something very honest and very kind which made my day: 'Mikyla, to be truthful I didn't like you before. Everyone was going on about you and how good you were, but I thought, I'm already in the show, what's the big deal about her? I've seen the stuff between you and Darren and it's good, really good. I don't want to work against you. From now on let's work as a team, all three of us.'

From that moment on he was adorable and we really did all work as a team.

The first episode of *Hollyoaks* that I was in was a very big episode because it featured Gary Lucy's character, Luke, getting raped. Everyone was invited to a screening of it in the set pub, the Dog in the Pond. I sat cross-legged on the floor with all the established cast. Gary was tremendous and deservedly won *Hollyoaks* its first Soap Award. I couldn't believe it when I saw myself come up on the screen. It's a very peculiar sensation, watching yourself. I cringed at the parts of my performance I thought could have been better, but also felt pleased with parts too.

Terri approached me and said, 'Babe, we're all going to Jalon's after the screening. Do you want to come along?'

'Oh, that would be great, but I'm looking very scruffy,' I said. Jalon's was an upmarket restaurant in Liverpool. 'Will everyone be getting dressed up?'

'Oh, no, babe. Come as you are, anything goes.'

But then I saw Terri change into a backless pink satin dress and decided not to go. I didn't want people to poke fun at me in my dowdy clothes.

Jalon's is now one of my favourite places on earth, and Terri was right – anything goes, and that's part of its charm. That place holds so many of my fondest memories. The menu is relatively simple and I order the same thing every time I go. The staff don't bother asking me any more. It's always pâté to start followed by a shoulder of lamb that is cooked to perfection – Gordon Ramsay, eat your heart out.

After the screening, everybody had rushed to congratulate Gary, who, at nineteen, had delivered an outstanding performance. He was surrounded by a sea of slim beautiful blondes, accompanied by several very good-looking guys. They were all so perfect I felt as if I was having an out-of-body experience. In my mind's eye, I could see how different I was and doubted that I would ever be able to integrate into this unrealistically attractive group of people. I hovered around awkwardly. Never having met Gary before, I was unsure of him. I made the assumption that most people do that if somebody is good-looking and famous AND talented, they are also likely to be arrogant, vain and egotistical, though in fact this wasn't the case with Gary. I decided that I should probably steer clear of him. As I stood there I looked around me, and thought, 'Well, girl, this is it, your fifteen minutes of fame. Take note because this could be as good as it gets.'

I was very unsure about what I should do and embarked on a frantic internal monologue in my head: Should I go and congratulate him, or is that trying too hard? Will he even recognise who I am? What if I go over there and they all start laughing? Ha, ha, look at the fat girl trying to be our friend. OK, so I can't risk that. Maybe I should say nothing and just go. But then I may appear rude. I'll just shout out a casual, 'Bye, guys.' But what if nobody answers and the producers see this and realise . . . *I don't fit in*?

I was saved from internal combustion from those conflicting arguments by Jimmy McKenna, who played Mr Osbourne, the landlord of the Dog in the Pond.

'All right, big 'un, congratulations – you were brilliant in that episode. I really hope they keep you on. I'm going to have a word with Phil Redmond about it. Are you coming along to Jalon's with us?'

I shook my head, but his comments cheered me up no end.

The feedback from other actors was also positive. I bumped into Lewis Emerick who played Mick Johnson from *Brookside* and he was equally enthusiastic. I felt more affinity with the *Brookside* actors, who were career actors, than with the *Hollyoaks* cast members, who were mainly career models. Despite my self-doubt about my ability to fit in socially with the *Hollyoaks* actors, I went home euphoric about the praise I had received for my acting ability. Maybe I'm going to make it after all, I thought.

13
A Case of a Pretend Boyfriend and a Suit of Armour

20 stone

Soon after I joined *Hollyoaks*, I was invited to the Soap Awards. I was sent the invitation through the post, and both my mum and I were ecstatic when it landed on the doormat. Without doubt this was the most thrilling event I'd ever been invited to. It was the proof I craved of the producers' intention to turn me into a fully fledged cast member. The thought of rubbing shoulders with stars in ballgowns sent an ecstatic shiver down my spine. Then I realised that I would have to find a ballgown. I couldn't show up looking like Cinderella. For most people, sorting out an outfit would be fun, especially with a £1,000 budget and a city full of clothes shops. Needless to say, this wasn't exactly how things went.

My mum and I trailed the length and breadth of the north-west of England with hugely disappointing results. Liverpool – 0, Manchester City Centre – 0, Manchester Trafford Centre – 0 and finally Leeds – 0. I didn't manage to net anything in a single one of these shopping Meccas. By the time we reached Leeds I was distraught and was about to give my Soap Awards ticket to the first bag lady I laid eyes on. 'There you go, love, enjoy yourself, won't ya!' I said in my head.

After six long hours we stumbled upon Ernest Jones, and as I had done over the years, I gazed longingly in the window at the Tag Heuer watches. After a couple of minutes drooling and discussing hypothetically which one to buy, we looked at each other and it all made sense. Without saying anything, we walked into the shop and I asked to try on the watch I'd set my heart on. It was beautiful and I fell in love with it immediately. I swear that it was made just for me, except that the watchmaker got bored halfway through and didn't put enough links in to accommodate my fat, ugly wrists. But that's just a minor detail and I wasn't going to let it deter me.

The jeweller kindly offered to add the links while we continued shopping.

'To hell with the shopping,' I said to my mum.

After that substantial purchase I needed a stiff drink. Having blown my entire budget, I was going to look like Cinders with no chance of making it to the ball. Or turn up naked except for a watch which I wasn't sure was what the producers had had in mind.

Where's my Fairy Godmother? I thought. If she does exist, now would be a very good time for her to appear.

It was only a week before the awards. The next day I had a session of pulling out every item of clothing I owned from my wardrobe, trying it on, gazing with loathing at myself in the mirror before discarding it in disgust. Sadly my life was frequently punctuated by those 'throwing clothes in a heap on the floor' sessions. They usually ended with me flinging myself face down on my bed and sobbing. I'd gained a few pounds since joining the cast of *Hollyoaks*. I was nowhere near my top weight of 24 stone 7 pounds, but I was hovering around the 20-stone mark, which didn't please me. There was a subsidised canteen at work, and cheap, fatty food was never a good thing to waft in front of my nostrils. Also, there was a local sandwich shop that I often frequented for lunch. There I requested a sandwich on wholemeal bread with cranberry sauce, turkey, bacon, avocado, cucumber, mayonnaise and black pepper in it. The sandwich became more famous than me locally, and the shop reported that customers were coming in asking for a 'Mikyla'.

It wouldn't have been possible for more things to have gone wrong at these first Soap Awards. I think I was doomed from the moment I received the invitation. I asked a tall, handsome, Scandinavian-looking actor friend called Danny to accompany me. We'd been friends for many years and were both disciples of David Johnson. I've never been attracted to blonds or actors, and he was no exception, but I secretly hoped people would assume we were a couple. I quite wanted them to think that an above-average specimen of a man had chosen to date somebody like me. Unfortunately, I would have been far better off inviting a less gorgeous male friend whom I could have had a good laugh with.

I ended up wearing a not-so-little black dress that had been in my wardrobe for donkey's years, but I reasoned that as nobody had made any adverse comments about it the last time I wore it (although they hadn't made any favourable ones either), I would at least feel comfortable. The dress had a slit up the leg, so of course there was waxing to be done and the issue of my white (almost-blue) skin. I used to ponder about whether the beautician doing my legs would be tempted to ask for double as my legs were twice the average size. I hadn't really thought about their colour, though, until the girl waxing them brought it up. As she ripped the fair hairs out of my plump thighs, she said, 'Are these on show?'

Rip. 'Arrgh . . . yes,' I gasped, my eyes watering with pain.

'Well, you better do something about the colour of them.' Rip.

Next thing I know I was booked in two days later to have the obligatory *Hollyoaks* tan applied from a bottle.

My skin turned a deep shade of orange. Horrified, I spent the next three days exfoliating, but it was all to no avail. I was terrified that I'd be scarred for life and the chemical tan took weeks and weeks to fade.

I booked into my local hairdresser's in Blackburn before the big night. I wanted to have natural-looking GHD-style curls, but again the plan went horribly wrong. My hairdresser didn't know what I was talking about when I asked for glamorous, natural-looking curls. Instead I emerged from the salon looking like a cross between Brian May and Annie.

When we met up at the station to go to London for the awards, Danny took one look at me and said unsympathetically, 'What on earth have you done to your hair? I like it much better the way you usually have it.'

We jumped on the train down to London, and when we arrived it was bucketing down with rain so we had to wait ages and ages for a cab. My invitation said to arrive at the awards ceremony by 5.15 p.m. I was panicking that we'd be late and would miss it. We'd been booked into the Grosvenor Hotel and arrived there looking like a pair of drowned rats. I gave my name and Danny's at reception. Humiliation of humiliations, they couldn't find me listed anywhere. There was a queue of people behind me and I felt like some sort of gatecrasher. Finally my name was located on the list. The receptionist almost shouted out, 'Double or twin?'

'Twin, please,' I said under my breath.

But even louder he asked, 'Sorry, madam, what was that? Double or Twin?'

I snapped back, 'Twin, please.' Now everyone in the queue would know their speculation had been correct and that this handsome hunk by my side was not my boyfriend.

When we got up to the room, we started fighting over who was going to use the bathroom first. Danny insisted that he should take priority. By this time I was nearly at breaking point.

'My hair is a mess, my fake tan has turned me into a laughing stock, and I haven't even started on my make-up, which, let's face it, is another disaster waiting to happen. And you honestly believe your need is greater than mine?'

He reluctantly conceded. I dived in there and turned on the shower. I was so keen to remove the sopping-wet clothing I'd been wearing for the last hour that I'd forgotten to take my evening outfit into the bathroom with me. Once I stepped out of the shower and unfolded the bath towel provided by the hotel, I realised it wouldn't even cover one of my legs, never mind the vast expanse of streaky orange flesh I wanted to hide. As I stood there pondering the best course of action, there was a knock at the door.

'How long are you gonna be? We've got to be down there in twenty minutes, and I can't be rushing or I'll end up looking a mess!'

I wanted to say, 'Oh, piss off. I've got more important things to worry about than the way you're gonna look,' but of course I didn't say that. 'Yeah, OK, I'll be right out,' I muttered.

Short of a needle and thread to stitch four towels together, I was going to have to put back on the water-drenched outfit that lay in a soggy heap on the bathroom floor. As I opened the door, I looked no different than I had ten minutes previously when I closed it, apart from the *Stars in Your Eyes*-style steam bellowing behind me.

'What the hell have you been doing in there? I thought you were having a shower,' Danny growled.

Unable to explain my apparent insanity, I just stepped aside and said, 'Do you want the bathroom or not?'

Fortunately his vanity overcame his curiosity and I was not forced to explain any further.

As I sat in my pyjamas struggling to even out my eye make-up and watching my frizzy fringe take shape as it dried, I started to think, They've invited me here just so they can have a really good laugh at me.

My paranoia was worsening by the minute. After a passable attempt at applying make-up, I attacked the rogue curls with industrial quantities of hairspray and managed to manipulate my hair into something remotely like a style.

Then it was time to climb into the most important part of my outfit – the re-enforced underwear that would attempt to give the effect of a reduced body size and shave at least one dress size, possibly two, off my frame.

The amount of temporary instant weight loss achieved is based solely on the wearer's capacity for discomfort and their pain threshold. Mine has always been quite high in this area. My feet, however, are a different story. I have zero tolerance for uncomfortable shoes and too much respect for my feet to abuse them. Let's not forget that those poor buggers used to carry around 24 stone 7 pounds and they never once complained. I could still hear the shower running, so figured it was safe to embark on this mission without being caught midway.

As a seasoned Lycra-wearer, I knew that putting the corsetry over my head was more effective than pulling it up. It's a gravity thing: starting at the bottom just pushes all the fat upwards, and by the time I've piled all that in, the bodice part has stretched outwards, making it shorter, so there is little space left for my ample boobs, which get dragged down. If you pull down, you can stop at the height you wish your boobs to sit, then scoop the unsightly bit up and fasten it between your legs with the poppers, which appear to have super powers and never come undone, despite the inhuman strain to which they're subjected.

I had got about a third of the way through this task, to the point where the garment is still twisted and needs unravelling at the back before my boobs are even in place, when I heard the shower stop. I then glanced down at the bed and saw Danny's suit laid out.

Realising I now only had the time it took him to wrap a towel round himself and unlock the door to sort myself out, I ended up putting my dress over the twisted body suit and folding my arms to conceal my lopsided breasts. As soon as he emerged from the steamed-up bathroom, I dived in there to struggle further with my straitjacket.

A while later I came out to find Danny still in his boxers. 'Come on, we need to get downstairs – we're already fifteen minutes later than the invitation specified!' I said agitatedly.

I was terrified that the cars ordered to take us from Park Lane to the BBC in White City would leave without us. 'Come on, Danny, come on!' I shouted.

'All right, keep your hair on,' he said casually in his strong Manchester accent.

By the time we made it downstairs, we were twenty minutes late and the foyer was deserted.

'Where the hell is everyone?' I said to Danny. 'They've gone without us – I knew this would happen.'

I was convinced all my efforts were a waste of time. I should have known I couldn't possibly get to go to an event like that. Nobody wants to see a fat bird trying to look like a film star. They would rather I was invisible.

Eventually I bumped into Ross Davidson, a lovely Scottish actor who played Andy Morgan, one of the parents in the show. He was still dressed in his jeans.

'How come you're not all dressed up?' I asked him. 'Am I missing something here?'

'Oh, did nobody tell you? The actual ceremony doesn't kick off for hours. They always tell people to come miles too early because we're usually ridiculously late and there are so many of us to organise,' he said. 'You can chill out for a while. There won't be even a whiff of an award for another three or four hours.'

I was hugely disappointed that I'd got myself massively

stressed out for nothing. Now I was all dressed up with quite literally nowhere to go. Danny had wandered off to check out the talent. I went back upstairs to my room. Impulsively I downed several miniature bottles of spirits and, bolstered by the alcohol, I returned to the foyer, which by now had filled up. Lots of people who I knew slightly didn't acknowledge me, which I found peculiar. If I was ever in a social situation where I knew people, I was always acutely aware of those who were new or shy or didn't know many people. I would try to pair them up with nice, friendly people who would include them in their conversations. I wished that someone would come and verbally scoop me up and enfold me in a circle of warm chatter. I hovered uncertainly on the edge of everyone else and wished I was anywhere but there, in the middle of a circus that didn't encourage elephants!

A few skinny girls said sympathetically to me, 'Oh, you look nice.'

'For a fat girl,' I added silently. I tried to smile and say thank you as graciously as I could. At times when I was dressed up nicely and felt good in my skin, I quite enjoyed being looked at, although I hated people staring. There was a fine line between the two, and tonight I felt that everyone was staring critically at me. I wished that an exceedingly large stone would appear that I could roll myself under.

After the award ceremony, I went back to the Grosvenor Hotel. Although I had only just started working on *Hollyoaks* and wasn't flush with cash, I offered to buy a round of drinks for a few people. The bill came to a shocking £97.

Gary Lucy had won an award for best newcomer for his role as a victim of male rape. Lisa Riley came over to us and gushed to Gary about his performance, but hardly acknowledged me. Later that evening, while Danny sulked in the hotel room because he had been unable to secure a woman to bed who looked as gorgeous as he did, I continued chatting to people in the bar. One woman, who was a hairdresser and girlfriend of an actor I didn't know, was particularly friendly towards me.

'I don't really know anyone here,' I confessed to her. 'I've only just joined *Hollyoaks* and I feel a bit out on a limb.'

'Oh, don't worry, you can stick with us,' she said, squeezing my hand. 'We'll be popping up to the room soon for a few drinks, but you're more than welcome to join us.'

'Oh, thanks, that would be wonderful,' I said gratefully. Anything not to look like I was a spare part, sitting all alone.

The three of us went up to their room and the man disappeared into the bathroom.

'Why don't you have a look in the minibar and fix us all some drinks?' she said, and smiled.

I obediently opened the fridge.

'How many?' her boyfriend called from the bathroom.

'Three,' she replied and disappeared into the bathroom. 'Pop into the bathroom,' she called. 'And bring the drinks.'

At that point I got an inkling that cocaine might be featuring. I wondered if soap stars really did use as much coke as the tabloids claimed they did.

She had been bending over doing her line. She straightened up and said, 'There you go, have one of these.'

I'd never tried cocaine and had never been particularly curious about it. But once it was presented to me, I decided I might as well have a go. Almost immediately I felt brighter. I had no idea then how much coke was in a gram and how many lines you could get out of that. I felt as if my nose was running after I'd snorted it, even though it wasn't.

We went back downstairs to join the others. I started to panic about the etiquette of cocaine use. Was I expected to invite them up to my room for a few reciprocal lines? I had no idea where on earth I'd be able to get hold of the drug. Instead I bought them some drinks and hoped they would suffice. Ironically it was the following day that all the tabloids were full of shock-horror shots of Danniella Westbrook's missing septum.

I wandered into that first Soap Awards with no clue of what sort of build-up was involved for the average cast member of a soap, but I stayed on at *Hollyoaks* and by my second year – 2001 – I had become an expert. The ceremony was in April, and from February onwards the actresses talked of little else.

'Who's making your outfit? Are you getting your legs waxed the day before, or the week before?'

In the run-up to the awards ceremony I would find sketches of glamorous frocks lying around the green room.

'I'm not sure whether to reveal my boobs, my midriff or my legs,' the girls said to each other, knowing that they were likely to look good revealing any combination of the three.

Meanwhile I wondered how much I needed to cover up so that I looked OK. While the women immersed themselves in girlie award talk, I chatted and joked with the crew, a down-to-earth bunch of Scousers. I realised that I felt much more at home in male company than female. I was treated as an honorary bloke by the crew and took this as a great compliment. I didn't expect anyone to rush to take my photo the first year of the awards because I had only just joined the cast of *Hollyoaks*, but the lack of interest in taking my picture on the red carpet in subsequent years was hurtful, even though part of me didn't want to be in the public eye.

The photographers never remembered my name, and as they peered through the lens at me, they lost interest when someone slimmer and lovelier sashayed up the red carpet. Although I wasn't craving publicity, I felt irked that I was an outsider purely because of my size. I knew that if I had been able to display a washboard midriff and pull a muscled Premier League footballer, all would be right between me and the paparazzi.

Some of my skinny counterparts were truly stunning, but some were just slim blondes with average faces who were prepared to flash a considerable amount of flesh. In my final year I had a stunning black corseted dress made for me, which gave me a lovely hourglass shape. The BAFTAs were a few weeks before the Soap Awards and we were only given a week's notice of our invitation so alas my corseted dress wasn't ready in time. The oh-so-perfect Trinny and Susannah sneered at my appearance, in their TV commentary. I'd lost over 3 stone by this point, although that wasn't apparent to them. I supposed I'd have to lose at least another six before I had any chance of receiving a favourable remark. They didn't refer to me by name but merely said, 'And as for the big girl, she'd do much better if she wore a corset rather than that shapeless sack.'

There's no right to reply with Trinny and Susannah, but I would have loved to have said, 'Actually, my corset is being crafted as we speak and you wait till you see me wearing it in a few weeks' time at the Soap Awards,' but I never had the satisfaction, and I don't suppose they would have been remotely interested in anything of a sartorial nature that I had to say.

14
If She's Fat, Then I Must Be Fat

22 stone

As I became more established on *Hollyoaks*, I got past my initial feelings of gratitude for being given some acting work and hankered after having a contract. After nine months they finally gave me one. Everyone got paid the same rate per episode, so the aim was to get into as many episodes as possible. I was offered twenty-five episodes a year, which really isn't very many. Some of the other cast members were offered a similarly small number. My agent was reluctant to argue for more and seemed to take the view that I should be grateful for what was offered.

So I raised it myself with Jo Hallows, the producer.

'To be honest, Jo, twenty-five episodes is £25,000 a year. I could earn that in any nine-to-five job and lead a normal life, and it really isn't worth staying for. I know the others who've been given twenty-five episodes feel the same way.' In truth the biggest problem is that most other cast members earn three times what you do, but you are expected to keep up with their spending. Everyone you come in contact with assumes that you earn a six figure salary.

Jo always listened carefully to what cast members had to say. She explained the reasoning behind it, and said that in order to promise me the same as the more established cast members, she would need to do the same for other people in my situation, which would take her over her annual quota and not leave room for new characters. But after ten minutes of negotiation I managed to secure five more episodes for all of us.

'Thank you very much, Jo.' I beamed. I felt I'd scored a significant victory.

With the exception of me, the actresses on *Hollyoaks* were hired for their blonde identikit looks and sylph-like figures. I was hired to play a fat girl, and my appearance remained reasonably consistent throughout my time on the show. One of the girls, however, who was hired as a slim blonde let herself go a bit and was pulled up by the producers and ordered to lose weight and cut down on her nights out on the town, which were affecting her looks.

Some of the cast members said, 'I bet Mikyla won't be too pleased to hear about that.' But actually I thought that the show's bosses were being perfectly reasonable in asking her to maintain the appearance she had when she was hired.

After the initial horror story with the wardrobe department for my first episode, my outfits did improve. My character, Chloe, was supposed to be fashionable and slightly kooky and so I didn't mind wearing things that I wouldn't have worn in real life, such as tight cropped pink jeans with a cerise cowboy hat. Again, though, I sometimes wondered if the outfits were crossing the line between quirky and laughing stock.

My relationship with the wardrobe department remained lousy. A couple of the staff put together flattering outfits for me, but most of them either couldn't be bothered or thought to themselves, She's fat so she'll look awful in anything we give her, so why bother?

Good wardrobe people and make-up artists say that it's part of their job to make the actors not just look good but feel good, but the bad ones barely consider that aspect of their work at all. When I was presented with unflattering outfits, I would often have a little rant to whoever happened to have the misfortune of being in the dressing room.

The dressing room was one big room with a toilet and shower cubicle in the corner, then a row of lockers – very reminiscent of a girls' changing room at school. It took me about six months to pluck up the courage just to get changed in there. When I first started, I would go into the toilet to change or pretend to send texts on my phone until the dressing room emptied. Most of the girls would get in, get changed and go straight on set, although there were one or two who liked to prance around in their underwear for half an hour. I often wonder if they sacrificed half an hour of extra sleep to arrive earlier and allow time to display their near-naked bodies before going on set.

Understandably I didn't want to wear clothes that made me look 3 stone heavier than I actually was, and in the end Jo Hallows gave me a budget to buy my own clothes for the show, something that was an enormous relief to me.

It's always easy to dress skinny girls and make them look good, but in case any budding fashion designers are reading this, here are a few tips that may not work for all large women but have certainly worked well for me: dresses are best avoided, as are trousers, which can ride up over a large belly, making the legs uneven. Tops and skirts work best, especially when teamed with knee-high boots, which can hide a multitude of sins. Long hair has an elongating effect, and it's always worth dazzling with cleavage. Upper arms should be hidden at all times, or at least have something draped around them if wearing a sleeveless evening outfit.

With my contract and the more satisfactory wardrobe arrangements, my confidence on *Hollyoaks* grew. When I had first begun working on *Hollyoaks*, I had lived at home. My mum had provided a Rolls Royce accommodation service and I loved being with her. Having said that, I was now almost twenty-three and knew that I really should be thinking about moving out, but I didn't want to upset her. My mum and dad had been talking for ages about moving to France, but my mum refused to budge until I was settled.

Ben Hull, one of the cast members who I got along very well with, offered me a room in a flat he was sharing with some of the other cast members – Gary Lucy and Terri Dwyer. I was very enthusiastic about moving in with the boys but had doubts about Terri, who they nicknamed 'Dame Dwyer'.

'I'd love to move in with you, Ben,' I said, 'but I'm not sure I'll get on with Terri.'

'Oh, Terri's all right, Mikyla, really she is,' said Ben.

I'm so glad I took his word for it, as that home provided me with a year of continual laughter and support. He explained that the main part of the house had four bedrooms and then there was a separate staircase leading to another bedroom and bathroom, which Terri had.

I moved in gradually, thinking that it would be better to prepare my mum bit by bit for the separation from the baby of the family. Surreptitiously I bought myself a TV, a bed and a music centre, and after a three-month 'breaking-in' period for my mum, I announced to her that I was moving out.

My mum accepted the move; my dad said very little about it. Mum taped my *Hollyoaks* shows, but I'm not sure that my dad ever watched an episode. Jay, Sam and Ella were pleased for my success on the show but all had very busy lives, and as far as I know none was a regular viewer. Sam had moved to France by now, Ella was still with Precious, and Jay kept on getting very impressive promotions in the army. Mum and Dad didn't move to France straight away but planned to.

Sharing a house with cast members was a wonderful experience, probably akin to university students living away from home for the first time, still flushed with idealism. They drank wine and I got into drinking wine too. After work we sat around drinking and talking about everything under the sun – love, sex politics, films. I loved every minute of it.

I felt very settled in the house and was happy with my new contract, but my position in *Hollyoaks* remained precarious. My scenes were often part of the 'comedy strand' of an episode and so if the writers needed more time for the core scenes, the easiest thing to drop was the comedy. I longed to have a storyline of my own, something that would elevate me beyond the status of jester and show that I could do serious stuff as well. I was fed up of being the chirpy, fat, funny bird from *Hollyoaks*. The trouble was, they didn't really know what to do with me. My first on-screen relationship fizzled out after about three months.

Then I started another relationship, which also only lasted for a few months. Then a young man called Kristian Ealey joined the soap. He was a savvy Scouser who Phil Redmond liked because he reminded him of his younger self. He had played the same character on *Brookside*, and when *Brookside* folded and Kristian moved over to *Hollyoaks*, it was the first time ever that a character had moved from one soap to another. The writers didn't know what to do with Kristian either, so they paired me up with him. I waited patiently for a few months but no sign of a storyline emerged. I knew that if I was slimmer and prettier, I would have been much busier on the soap, which after all was a vehicle for beautiful people. Although I knew that I was a well-liked member of the cast, I often felt like second best because of my size. At the time some of the people who'd been hired for their model looks were weak actors, and I was becoming increasingly frustrated that because I didn't look like them, I wasn't getting the opportunity to show what I could do. I would have liked to have been involved in a dramatic storyline that had nothing to do with my weight, but knew that that was unlikely to happen. So I decided to suggest a storyline myself, and opted for a theme that I knew the producers were much more likely to go for.

I took a deep breath and came straight out with it: 'What do you think about a storyline about my weight?' I said to Charlotte, one of the producers.

Her eyes widened. 'Is that something you'd feel comfortable about doing, Mikyla?' she asked.

'Yes, I would, and I think it's something that could strike a chord with lots of the teenage girls who watch *Hollyoaks* and feel uneasy about their bodies.'

'Well, I'm not sure that's something the viewers would feel comfortable with,' she said.

'Yes, but it's not just about being fat. It's about self-esteem and self-image, and that can apply to anyone who feels different. In real life people do make cruel comments about people who are fat or different in some way, and we could reflect that reality in a storyline.'

Charlotte went away and discussed it with the other producers and writers. She got back to me very quickly. 'Mikyla, everybody's keen, so let's go for it,' she said.

Jo was particularly enthusiastic. Kaddy Benyon was one of the writers who was going to be working on my storyline. She was excellent at her job and had written great comedy scenes for me. I looked forward to seeing how she would put together something more serious. She herself was over-weight and felt that my weight should not be an issue.

'Why do we need to cover this at all?' she asked the producers. 'Why can't Chloe just be the great person that she is?'

'But it was Mikyla who suggested this,' said Jo Hallows. 'She says that it's patronising not to refer to her size. In real life it would be a point of conversation, so this is something she feels really strongly about.'

Kaddy raised her eyebrows but offered no further objections. She knuckled down to writing my storyline and couldn't have produced anything more perfect. My story began when my character, Chloe, was standing for election as student president at college. Chloe played an important role in college life – she ran the radio station and was its agony aunt, and she fronted safer-sex campaigns and warned people about the dangers of contracting sexually transmitted infections. My character was happy, funny and positive, and the writers knew they couldn't turn me into a sad, depressed figure overnight, that it all had to happen gradually as the result of a series of blows.

Chloe fully expected to be elected as student president. She was a campaigner who had demonstrated a commitment to fighting for justice and to acting in the interests of the students. The writers used a character called Jamie to undermine Chloe. He found out that one of her earlier nicknames was 'Chloe Bruce the Moose' and he drew moose antlers on to all the pictures of her on her campaign posters and turned her into a complete laughing stock.

Jamie was standing against Chloe for election and all he promised the students was cheaper beer. It transpired that he had absolutely no commitment to the job or the students but had found out that the post of president came with free accommodation. Desperate to secure a rent-free place, he came up with the plan to sabotage Chloe's chances of being elected. Once she lost the election, she started to analyse herself very critically and decided that she wasn't worthy of winning. Kristian Ealey now played Chloe's boyfriend Matt: he stuck by her and tried to cheer her up, but nothing worked. Chloe had decided that she disliked herself so much that there was no possible way anyone could love her.

I got on well with most of the directors, but when we did this story I got into an argument with one of them. I found that, generally speaking, the directors who had previously been actors were much more empathetic towards the needs of the actors and more prepared to enter into discussions about alternative ways to do scenes. The director I got into the disagreement with had not been an actor.

In one scene Chloe had bought eight little pots of fromage frais and had reasoned with herself in the shop that she would only eat one and save the others for the rest of the week. But in that episode it showed her returning again and again to the fridge, hating herself more, then reaching for yet another pot of fromage frais and eating it. The director wanted me to down all the pots in one, like vodka shots, but I refused.

'No, that isn't how it works with food. It's about trying to resist the grip of this hopeless addiction and failing miserably,' I said.

'But the shot would look much better if you downed them all in one go,' said the director.

'Yes, but it wouldn't be real, it wouldn't be how it is,' I argued.

'Just do as you are told,' he thundered. 'I'm the director.'

Although the director was supposed to have the last word, I was determined not to concede this point. I wasn't interested in him getting a stunning shot at the expense of the authenticity of the scene.

'I haven't put my heart and soul into the storyline for the last three months to have it all rubbished in one scene just so you can get the shot you want,' I argued.

'This is what happens when actors are allowed to do storylines about themselves,' he muttered.

My heart was pounding with frustration.

'This storyline isn't about me. It's about self-image,' I said. 'It's something that many viewers will be able to relate to, whatever their hang-ups are. A lot of the teenage girls who watch the show feel this awful pressure that they won't become successful adults unless they're perfect and beautiful. There's an important message for them in this. Don't you understand?'

I went to see one of the producers and ranted. 'I'm sorry but I'm not prepared to do the scene that way. Thousands of viewers have identified with how fatness is lived out in daily life. Swigging the fromage frais almost simultaneously will not ring true with anyone who has experienced anything approaching what Chloe is experiencing.'

I felt a huge moral responsibility to get this right. People used to and still do come up to me in the street and say how much they love Chloe because of her imperfections. Her flaws make her a person they can relate to. It was as if everyone else in the cast was too perfect to have any resonance with ordinary viewers. The storyline showed that Chloe hadn't changed but when things changed around her it had a profound effect on her. In the end I got my way and the scene was shot in a manner that I knew was true to people who desperately tried but repeatedly failed to control their food intake.

Just before we were due to shoot a key scene in which Chloe rejected his heartfelt proposal of marriage, Kristian said to me, 'I know what a big scene this is for you, Mik, and I promise I'll work on it and we'll nail it on the day. I won't let you down.'

'Thanks,' I said. 'That means a lot.'

As he uttered words of love to Chloe, working up to his big proposal, he was shouted down by her. She grabbed rolls of loose flab from her midriff and half shouted, half cried, 'Don't patronise me. You don't love this. Don't lie to me. Why don't you go and find someone else who isn't so disgusting to look at?'

He said, 'But I love you – none of that matters to me.'

'Don't lie,' came Chloe's sharp response.

In the end she succeeded in driving away the man she loved. A perfect, self-destructive act.

On the day of filming we were the first scene of the day. I'd struck a deal with Alistair, one of the directors. I knew I was one of his favourites and vice versa. I negotiated with him before the shoot day and we agreed that if my performance was strong enough we would film the three-and-a-half-minute scene in one shot with no breaks or editing. It would be shot as one continuous moment. As much as he liked me, he wasn't prepared to promise, but we could try.

Most of the crew by this point knew about our bargain so pulled out all the stops to ensure there were no technical glitches to jeopardise my performance. There was a real buzz on set. Everybody milled around doing their bit. It was by this point 9.30 a.m. and we were running behind.

The scene was very emotional and I gave it my all. There was anger, followed by shame, followed by tears and plenty of snot. Kristian performed beautifully, which made the whole thing even more touching.

As the director called, 'Cut,' the crew downed tools and clapped. That was totally unprecedented. It wasn't just for me; it was for everybody involved. Between us we'd nailed it. I raced upstairs to watch the scene played back. I was still crying but was smiling at the same time.

'Well, will it hold? Please say yes, please.' I looked imploringly at Alistair.

After a long pause he said, 'Oh, piss off, you silly cow – of course it will.'

I was absolutely thrilled. This was the peak of my storyline and it was deeply personal to me.

There were many differences between me and Chloe, but during this time I felt that she was the only person in the world who related to me. Chloe was five years younger than me and was very similar to the way I had been at that age – much less sure of myself, and unconfident about which way to move forwards in the world. Chloe became my friend. I said 'good morning' to her every morning when I woke up and liked the familiarity of inhabiting her skin.

I learnt a lot on *Hollyoaks* and one thing was that nobody has a perfect face and body, even the women I assumed did from seeing them at a distance. Everyone has their own hang-ups and learns how to dress and do their make-up in a way that flatters them most. I knew how to dress cleverly so that I looked attractive in my clothes, but there was nothing that could be done to make my naked body look better. When I stood naked, my nipples almost touched my belly button and fat pooled over my hipbones, concealing them. I knew that I could make myself appear sexy with the right outfit, make-up and accessories, but naked, forget it. I made sure I kept men at arm's length so as not to shatter the clothed illusion of myself.

Another of the emotional scenes we did showed Chloe standing wrapped in a towel gazing at herself in disgust in the mirror. I was back up to 22 stone at the time. Then she allowed the towel to slip off her. The camera panned cleverly so as not to show all of me but enough to convey Chloe's disgust with her body.

I had expected it to be hard to act out such sensitive material, but I hadn't expected the experience to be quite as gruelling as it turned out to be. Although Chloe wasn't me, it was obviously a role that had enormous personal resonance, and taking that home every night became more and more difficult. If an actress plays a rape victim, it's emotionally draining, but when they go home at the end of the day, they aren't a rape victim. Chloe was in despair about her oversized body with rolls of fat slurping over the waistband of her clothes. When I went home at the end of the day, I still had to deal with those rolls of fat – I couldn't shed them like a fat suit and become somebody else. I was determined to remain cheerful during filming, but that made coping with the role much harder for me. I was acting a role of hating my body but pretending to like myself when the cameras stopped rolling. I didn't hate myself as much as Chloe hated herself, but the storyline brought up lots of difficult issues for me about my size and my perception of myself.

I received hundreds of supportive letters from viewers, overwhelmingly from women but a few from men too. One woman wrote that she had been beaten up in the street for being fat.

It was a very peculiar time for me because while I was getting lots of praise from viewers, cast members and crew for my performance, the storyline made me feel increasingly vulnerable.

I had always drunk quite a lot but now I drank more than ever in a bid to put as much space between Chloe and me at the end of each day as possible. I was getting through about three-quarters of a bottle of vodka every night. I woke up every single day with a hangover and stopped noticing that I felt as if I'd been hit with a sledgehammer.

I generally spent Sundays lying on the sofa all day after a couple of nights of drinking and taking cocaine and not sleeping. The most I managed to do was load up the washing machine. I also upped my consumption of junk food, mainly because I was working fourteen-hour days, and grabbed whatever food was closest to hand rather than taking time to plan healthy meals.

I managed to hide the emotional fallout that the storyline was having on me while I was at work. I was terrified that if I kicked up any sort of fuss I might be seen as a prima donna instead of good-sport, down-to-earth Mikyla. Hiding my true feelings put a lot of extra pressure on me. The storyline lasted for about three months. In the end Chloe regained a sense of perspective and tentatively began to get on with her life again.

After the enormous amount of emotion that I'd invested in turning the magnifying glass on myself, I felt very deflated. When Chloe sorted herself out and the angst faded away, I decided that I really should do something about my weight. In the two and a half years I'd been at *Hollyoaks* I'd gradually put on about 2 stone. I felt that emotionally I was running on empty. I felt that the weight storyline had turned such a spotlight on me that I had lost my sense of self. I no longer knew who I was. While the specific amount of weight that I'd gained wasn't the thing that distressed me, the more general issue of being large did. I decided that losing weight would give me a much-needed boost and help me regain my sense of identity.

15
Richard and Judy

22 stone

As the storyline about Chloe's weight issues aired, there was a flurry of media interest, including *Richard and Judy*. At first I was jumping for joy. The couple are daytime TV legends, but when I really started to think about it, I became apprehensive. I wasn't sure if they were 'Hollyoaks-friendly' and feared they may ridicule the show or, worse still, me. The subject of the slot on their show was food addiction. I was worried that it might be an extended mickey-taking exercise at the expense of fat people. As I travelled down to London first class on the train, various different scenarios played out in my head. I vowed that I would be very vigilant and avoid any of the obvious traps they might lay for me. I wanted to get across on the show how deeply hurtful people's remarks about weight could be and how much anguish they could cause to people like me who were already beating themselves up about their weight.

I arrived and wasn't sure what to do about announcing myself. To my surprise and relief, people seemed to know who I was. I never, ever thought of myself as famous. I was thrilled when I was shown to my dressing room.

'Oh, Ian McKellen was here yesterday,' added the production assistant casually.

'Ian McKellen, really.' I felt quite overwhelmed by the sheer famousness of the ground I was stepping on. Then I found a generous bunch of ruby-red amaryllis bound with hessian and a range of Molton Brown toiletries. I couldn't quite believe that they were for me. 'Are you sure these are for me?' I asked the assistant doubtfully.

'Of course they are: guests' perk,' said the assistant.

At that moment a researcher knocked on the door. 'Now, I'd just like to run through a few things with you,' she said. 'I understand you're a trained sumo wrestler. How would you feel about demonstrating some sumo wrestling on Richard?'

'Oh, no, absolutely not,' I said. Of all the scenarios I'd endlessly played out in my head, this one had never even featured as a distant speck on the horizon.

I looked at the press officer from *Hollyoaks* who had accompanied me. She shrugged. 'It's up to you, Mikyla.'

I saw numerous opportunities for exploitation if I allowed myself to be drawn into some kind of 'tussle for laughs' exchange.

The researcher could see that this was a non-negotiable situation and backed off. 'OK, no worries, I won't pursue that,' she said.

After that little bombshell I was definitely on the back foot. I wondered if there were any other tricks they might dream up for me and was very wary when I was installed on the sofa with a beaming Richard and Judy.

'So, Mikyla, you're doing a storyline in *Hollyoaks* about

obesity. That must be very personal to you,' said Richard. 'How do you feel about that storyline?'

'It was my idea,' I said proudly.

'Really? And what made you decide to suggest it?' asked Richard.

I was surprisingly relaxed about the fact that the show was live. 'I think it's a very important issue. It's not just about being overweight, it's the whole issue of self-image.'

'It seems that you've always embraced your size. It says here you used to work in Evans Outsize Shop?'

'They actually don't call it the "Outsize Shop" any more. It doesn't project the right image, so it's just called Evans.'

Straight away Richard flashed a look at Judy. 'You told me it was called Evans Outsize.'

Judy widened her eyes and through slightly gritted teeth said, 'Yes, well, obviously times have changed.' I let out a raucous laugh.

There was a hissing in their ears from the floor manager telling them that it was time to move on to the next guest, but Judy simply took her earpiece out and carried on talking.

'Do you see yourself as a positive role model for others?' asked Judy.

'I'm not saying that big is beautiful, or that being over-weight is the best thing in the world. What I'm saying is that it's not such a big deal,' I replied.

'And what do you make of Sophie Dahl's weight loss?'

Great question, Richard, I thought. I'm going to answer this one carefully.

I replied, 'I think it's a shame, as she made her name from being different, but ultimately it's about how you feel in yourself, so if she wasn't happy the way she was, then fair play to her.' There were at this point a couple of beads of sweat on my face.

'Very diplomatic,' said Richard, smiling.

I thoroughly enjoyed myself on the show. They made me feel incredibly relaxed, as if I was sitting in their front room having coffee with them.

As I walked off the set, one of the researchers said, 'Bloody hell, they liked you – you were supposed to be on for six and a half minutes but they kept you on for eleven. Are you going to stay behind for after-show drinks?'

'Oh, yes, absolutely, I'd love to,' I said.

Joe Pasquale was also a guest on the show and his time was cut because mine ran over. 'I only got three minutes because of you,' he said in mock annoyance.

'I'm so sorry,' I said.

We then went on to talk about diet and weight loss, which is always a conversation that makes me chuckle when it's with the opposite sex. I think women including myself often treat fat as a feminist issue and it's not. It just so happens that the media is far more obsessed with the size of the female physique than it is with the male.

At the beginning of 2006 I was invited back on to the show to go head to head with someone who had written an article in a newspaper about finding the sight of fat people offensive. I received a very effusive welcome from Richard and Judy.

'You're looking fabulous,' said Richard. Then a picture of me at my heaviest flashed up on the screen. 'Now that you've lost weight, how do you feel about that picture?' asked Richard.

'Well, aesthetically I know I look better now,' I said. 'But at the time I was happy with how I looked. I just made the best of myself.'

The man who had written about not liking to be around fat people seemed rather less opinionated in my presence. I think he felt he was the bad guy, while I was receiving plenty of support from Richard and Judy.

'In my home town there are lots of very overweight people. I see them stuffing chips into their mouths and I don't like to see it,' he said.

'Well, not everyone likes to look at older, balding men,' I said.

Richard roared with laughter.

'Derogatory comments just demoralise people who are overweight and make them reach for the biscuit tin,' I said. 'What people need is support and sound nutritional advice. It's important to be constructive.'

At the end of the interview Judy said, 'I want to say again how stunning you look, Mikyla. You so remind me of Sophie Dahl.'

'Thank you.' I beamed. 'Maybe I'll get the modelling contract and pots of money just like her.'

It is very intriguing to experience the show first hand. It's a very well-oiled machine that has an amazing understanding of what their audience wants. It's easy to assume that what they do is simple as they appear to breeze through it, but I'm sure the reality is far from it.

16
Don't Do Running

21 stone 7 pounds

Although Chloe had regained her confidence and moved on, I was feeling less upbeat, and the weight question continued to prey on my mind. I railed against prejudices towards fat people – the insulting comments, the assumption that we're all somehow inferior to thin people, the conviction that we have no control over ourselves and that if any negative event happens in our life that we'll automatically take refuge in binging. I also knew that I genuinely did not aspire to being a size 10 and did not believe that was where happiness lay. And yet . . .

Something wasn't right. There was no pressure on me at *Hollyoaks* to slim down. I knew I was valued there for what I could do, not what size my trousers were, but I was experiencing a deepening dissatisfaction within myself. I decided that losing weight so that I could fit into clothes more comfortably, walk up a flight of stairs more easily and no longer attract hard stares in the street would be extremely nice.

I'd dieted before, and when I had the time I still went on the exercise bike, so I knew that losing weight was achievable. I pondered what the best way to do it would be. The ever-inspiring Jo Hallows came up with a perfect solution.

Jo had invited Gary Lucy, who had by now left the show, Nick Pickard, who plays Tony, Jimmy McKenna and me to the Royal Television Society Awards. All of them were amongst my favourite people in the world and I had a wonderful time.

As we sat at our table, I said to Jo, 'You know, since doing the weight storyline in *Hollyoaks*, I've really been thinking seriously about trying to lose some.'

'Really?' said Jo.

'Yes, I'm not actually happy with myself at this weight. That storyline has really taken its toll on me.' Jo looked thoughtful.

A couple of days later she said, 'How would you feel about making a documentary about your weight loss as a sort of companion piece to the *Hollyoaks* storyline? We haven't got much money but we'd give you a director, Will, and when we sell the documentary, then you'll get some money.'

'That sounds perfect,' I said eagerly. 'It'll give me just the boost I need to make some changes in my life.'

I knew that being filmed would give me an incentive and would make me more competitive with myself about reaching certain goals. I was delighted that they had chosen Will, who was a friend as well as a producer and director. He understood me well and I got along excellently with him.

They advertised for a personal trainer to take me in hand and said that they would draw up a shortlist of applicants but that I could make the final choice. I asked my friend Nick Pickard what he thought of the idea.

'Well, it will put you under an awful lot of pressure, Miky, but I think you should go for it – it could be a great opportunity for you.'

The interviews with the personal trainers were interesting. They took place in a coffee bar above a swimming pool. It was the height of summer and was very hot. I had rivers of sweat running down my scalp and forehead.

I rejected the body builder, who was far bigger than me, because I was terrified he would bulk me up until I looked like him. I rejected the size-16 woman, who said she wanted to use the opportunity to shed weight herself, and the size-6 woman with a washboard stomach kitted out in Reebok and Nike from head to toe, even though she brought along with her a testimony from a client who she had helped go from a size 20 to a size 10. And then a cheeky man called Dave with his hair gelled into twists appeared. The banter between us began immediately.

'You're far too old to have your hair in that style,' I quipped. He acknowledged that I was right.

'What would you do if halfway through a training session I said, "I don't want to do any more, I want to go and have an ice cream."'

All the other trainers had replied, 'I would say, "You're doing so well, don't let yourself down."'

Dave said, 'I'd stop what we were doing immediately and say, "If that's what you want, then go and knock yourself out – have four ice creams, I couldn't care less. Just call me when you're ready to lose weight."'

Well, that was exactly the way to deal with my nonsense. He was hired on the spot. He had a motivated, sincere way of talking that appealed to me and immediately I knew that he was the one. He was ex-army and had the same 'can-do' attitude as my brother, Jay.

He began by doing an initial fitness check on me so that he would have a baseline to measure my progress against.

'In a year's time your fitness levels will have changed beyond recognition,' he said confidently.

First he set me to work on the treadmill with a heart-rate monitor and then he measured how long it took for my heart rate to return to normal after the exertion – the quicker the rate returns to normal after exertion, the fitter you are.

'Now, could you try and touch your toes for me.' He looked at me doubtfully, presuming that a person of my size would find such a task impossible. But in fact I managed it with ease. 'That's excellent, really excellent,' he said. 'We'll have you running in no time.'

I looked at him in horror. 'Oh, no you won't, I don't do running. It makes me look hideous: I bounce around all over the place. Don't ever ask me to run.'

I knew that I sounded aggressive, but I was terrified that if anyone caught sight of me running, with big pillows of vibrating flesh forming a 360-degree blanket around my hips, bottom and stomach, they would roar with laughter.

'Well, we'll see about that. Another thing you need to do is give up smoking. You won't be able to make much headway with improving your fitness levels with cigarettes damaging your lung capacity all the time.'

I gave him another filthy look. 'Oh, no, absolutely not. I can't give up eating, smoking and do all this exercise at the same time. You're asking too much of me.'

Dave told me later that he went home to his girlfriend

that night and said, 'I think I've bitten off more than I can chew here.'

I found out later that he was bipolar and had got involved in personal training to get the endorphin buzz from exercise and the fulfilment of helping people. He became involved in producing capsules of EPA fish oil, which have been proven to help with a range of conditions from ME to Huntingdon's disease and depression.

It's not something I'm proud to admit, but I know that I'm a bit spoilt. I don't deal well with the 'no' scenario. But once I started training with Dave, my competitive streak kicked in. Dave would ask me to do twenty sit-ups in the hope that I would manage fifteen, but I forced myself on.

If you want twenty sit-ups, you'll get twenty sit-ups, I thought, clenching my eyes and my jaws with exertion.

Sometimes when he asked me to do something tough, I said, 'Are you kidding me?' but I always did it.

As I puffed and panted through the weeks at the gym, finding that some things got easier although others didn't, my attitude towards exercise started to change. Instead of seeing it as an enormous chore and a mountain too high to climb, I began to look at my sessions at the gym in the same way that I would look at a pedicure – as a treat for my body. Lifting weights, doing sit-ups and star jumps and heaving the rowing machine backwards and forwards simply became part of my beauty regime. Will, the director, filmed hours and hours of footage. It wasn't only about my fitness and weight-loss programme, but about what it's like to be a fat person in a world that reveres thinness.

Dave explained to me various technicalities relating to weight loss that had previously been mysteries to me. 'You have to find what your heart rate needs to be in order to burn fat. If you don't exert yourself enough, you won't burn fat.'

He worked out that my ideal fat-burning zone was when my heart rate climbed to between 135 and 165 beats per minute. As I became fitter, brisk walking on the treadmill was no longer challenging enough to raise my heart rate to the required level.

Sneakily I began to run on the treadmill when Dave wasn't there. That boosted my heart rate and didn't make me look as ridiculous as I'd once feared. At last I decided to confess my U-turn to him.

'Er, Dave, I've got something to tell you,' I said one morning when he set about tilting the treadmill so it was on an incline to make the power-walking harder for me. 'For the last couple of weeks I've actually been running on the treadmill and I've survived!'

'Oh, have you now?' He grinned. 'I wondered how long it would take.'

Dave was right about the smoking too. A few months after we started I had given up, and like the running, it did boost my fitness. I also modified my eating habits, cutting down on fats and completely cutting out sugary alcohol.

I loved the filming. I wandered into shops like Etam and chatted to the shop assistants who were selling plus-size clothes. After their initial bashfulness in the presence of the camera, they began chatting away. I do have the gift of the gab and the shop assistants quickly seemed to feel relaxed in my company.

'Why is it that when they make clothes in a size eighteen they have the same styles that they have in a size ten?

Miniskirts and Lycra tops just aren't a good look when you're a size eighteen, no matter how much material they use.'

The plus-sized assistants nodded their heads vigorously in agreement with me.

'They're obviously not designed by plus-sized people,' giggled one assistant. 'No one who had ever struggled to get a Lycra top and teeny skirt over size-eighteen hips would design something like that.'

Part of the documentary involved asking my friends and family about my weight. It was important to see how they viewed me and if they thought I could or even should lose weight. We would then revisit them after a year and discuss my new figure and attitude to food and drink. My mum was very defensive about my size and refused to make any negative comments because she didn't want to hurt my feelings. Sarah Jones (Suranne) gave an insight into my relationship with clothes and the difficulty I have finding things I like that flatter me. She spoke of occasions when I had flatly refused to come to fabulous showbiz parties just because I couldn't settle on an outfit. Having also seen me at my biggest, she was confident I would be successful and looked forward to the new phase that this change of lifestyle would bring.

'I'm sure losing weight will banish some of Mikyla's demons,' she said.

Next to be interviewed was Gary Lucy, who I had shared a house with, along with the adorable Ben Hull, who played Lewis. Also my good friend Terri Dwyer and another skinny blonde who shall remain nameless.

When you live with people, it either makes or breaks

your friendship, rather like the friends students make at university. To this day I still have a strong relationship with all the people I mentioned, and they are some of my dearest friends. Gary and I became like brother and sister. He is one of my most valued friends and couldn't be further from the stereotype I assumed he was when I first met him.

It wasn't until I'd lost the weight that I was allowed to see the content of the interviews. It was very emotional to watch them. Gary's shocked me the most. Unlike the others, I had no idea what he was going to say. He was very protective of me in a brotherly fashion.

'I don't know why she has decided to do this,' he said. 'I think she is perfect just the way she is. That may sound cheesy, but it's true. I have every faith she'll succeed. I just hope she is doing this for herself and not to please anyone else, because she doesn't need to.'

I had tears rolling down my face as I watched the tape. They were all honest and supportive – that's why they're such wonderful friends.

Last to be interviewed was my brother. In the last few years Jay had made a complete turnaround from the days of taunting me about my weight and making me feel that the bigger I was, the less important I was as a human being. Even before I landed the role in *Hollyoaks* he had started to accept me as I was and relented about some of his earlier behaviour.

He was man enough to admit the error of his ways and made amends with me. I know that that made Ella very happy, as she hated to see any of us fall out or hear us make negative comments about each other.

Jay's interview was frank and open. He admitted that I had proved him wrong on numerous occasions and he conceded that fat people are not always miserable, unsuccessful slobs but can be happy, successful individuals – it just usually depended on their mindset, not their appearance. He said that some of his previous taunts had been an attempt at tough love, and some were reflective of his own weight battle and continued commitment to exercise in order to keep the flab at bay. During the interview he suggested that if I lost enough weight, I would be able to do a tandem parachute jump attached to him (one of his many physical pursuits). This did make me smile. I know it was meant to be the ultimate in encouragement, but for me it was a strong argument against losing a single pound!

Doing the documentary forced me to take the terrifying step of enrolling at a gym. I imagined these places to be full of honed, Lycra-clad skinnies, and never dreamt that I could possibly fit in. I conducted some car-park surveillance of various establishments, checking out the clientele who went in and out. Some seemed to be used by the prim and perfect types I feared, but not all. In the end I found one where people of all shapes and sizes went to work out, many of them in scruffy old tracksuits rather than in the latest gear. After my initial terror – stepping over the threshold for the first time felt worse than my first day at school – I found that I did fit in there and enjoyed exercising.

Unfortunately, despite my success in losing weight and the fact that I had continued starring in *Hollyoaks*, the documentary never saw the light of day, but Dave and I continued training together until I finished working on *Hollyoaks* and moved down to London. Although it was hard losing weight, Mersey TV didn't really push the documentary, and I wondered if it was because I wasn't going to transform into a clone of the other girls and would still be overweight at the end. I never got paid for it, but could argue that I actually got something much more valuable – I lost 3 stone 8 pounds and kept it off.

The things I learnt while working with Dave are still precious to me today and very much guide when and how I exercise. He also helped me to enjoy the physical activity for its own sake. If I don't exercise, I get emotionally very low. Every so often I rebel and say I'm tired or am feeling a little under the weather, so take a few days off from the gym. Within a week I'm tearing my hair out and could cry at the drop of a hat. I think all that stuff about endorphins must be right. Exerting myself physically gives me a sense of achievement and makes me feel strong inside and out. I swear I feel much better equipped to deal with what the world throws at me.

Thanks to Dave and the documentary, I'd lost a huge chunk of my body and its appearance had changed beyond recognition. For the first time I had firm bits otherwise known as muscles. You could see my legs were very defined and appeared to go on for ever. My arms, which had been weak and flabby, became firmer from doing so much boxing and sticking to the weight-training programme Dave had set. I became so much more interested in clothes and men, probably because both were more available than they had been previously. People commented that I had become quite 'girlie' – a first for me. I was a size 18 to 20 and felt healthy, more positive, not to mention desirable and even sexy. I had embarked on a new stage of my journey.

17
'He Practically Raped You'

18 stone 2 pounds

I knew that my time at *Hollyoaks* wouldn't last for ever – stars were written out all the time – but I kept hoping that I could put off the inevitable. Characters who were part of a family had much more chance of longevity on the show than singletons like me. It was harder to explain away the sudden absence of a group of four or five characters than it was to dispose of one person who wasn't tethered to blood relations, but they kept me on.

As I had become more established on the soap, I had begun to hang out with a group of people who used a lot of cocaine. Conveniently one of them was a dealer. In the year after my initial experience with the drug at my first Soap Awards, I had only used cocaine once or twice when it was offered to me at parties. Then I started to use it a few times a week. I learnt how to take it so that it heightened the effects of alcohol, how to take it to 'straighten me out' when I started to feel too drunk and how to try to avoid that greedy craving for more and more that was inevitably followed by the unpleasant flatness of the comedown. I didn't always succeed. At the second Soap Awards that I attended, I drank an enormous amount of alcohol and snorted copious amounts of coke. The following morning I felt too ill to move. Every cell in my body ached and pain bounced around the inside of my head, banging roughly against my skull.

But even when I was using large quantities of cocaine, I stuck to a few rules to keep my habit at least partially in check. I never used it alone, or when I was sober, or at work. There is so much talk of drugs within the modelling world you would have assumed that the other girls in the show would have been indulging, but the truth is, I was the only one who took drugs. The model types hit the gym, didn't really drink a great deal and steered clear of anything illegal. They were so clean-living that skipping the odd meal was their only vice.

Not long before I left the show, I sat down and attempted to work out how much money I'd spent on this recreational habit. Once I reached the thousands I stopped working it out. I couldn't bear to think about what else I could have spent the money on.

Despite my excessive use of this drug, I believed that most of the time I was using it I remained in control. On one traumatic occasion, though, this wasn't the case.

While I was working on *Hollyoaks*, I and other cast members would often go to hotels in different UK cities at weekends for parties and other social gatherings. My (dubious) reputation was growing as a person who could generally be relied upon to have some coke. We were staying in a hotel in Manchester, and some other friends were staying in a different hotel. We'd been partying in my room, but everyone had gone, and feeling very woozy, I had got into my pyjamas and was about to get into bed.

Suddenly there was a knock on the door. Standing there was a friend of a friend of mine. He was a man who was part of our circle but who I had never liked very much. He often used to look past me when he was talking to me, scanning the room to see if anyone better had arrived.

He walked into my hotel room and said, 'All right?' without seeming very interested in my response. I nodded but felt uneasy. He sat down in the chair while I perched stiffly on the edge of the bed.

'What are you doing here?' I said.

He shrugged and started fiddling with the TV.

'I haven't got any coke,' I added, to underline how unnecessary it was for him to be in my room.

'Anything good on the telly?' he said casually.

The last thing I wanted to do was see what was on the TV. 'I wouldn't know. It's late and I'm usually in bed by now,' I said, praying that he would take the hint. I felt a growing sense of unease.

'What have you got in your minibar?' he asked, sticking his head in the fridge.

I didn't like the way he was behaving and felt very uncomfortable, but he hadn't done anything unreasonable or outrageous enough for me to kick him out of the room.

He rummaged around, found some vodka and poured himself some. He didn't ask me if I wanted anything but just plonked himself on a chair in the middle of the room.

'Are you tired?' he asked.

'Yes, actually, I'm ready for turning in.'

'Well, don't let me stop you.'

'I think you should go now,' I said.

'Oh, it's a bit late for me to go back to my hotel now,' he said in a false friendly manner.

I was now starting to get a picture in my head of how this was going to play out, but I wondered if my imagination had run wild because the alcohol or the coke had made me paranoid.

'It'll only take you a few minutes if you jump into a cab,' I said, hoping to make that sound like an enticing option for him.

He didn't seem impressed with that suggestion. 'Why don't you get yourself to bed?' he said. His voice sounded very calm and measured.

I knew by this point that something unpleasant was about to happen. I was terrified but could see no way out. I felt like a sheep being circled by a wolf. A sheep would have made a run for it, but fear was quite literally paralysing me. My brain wanted to escape, but my body felt heavier than lead. I couldn't move. At the same time self-deprecating thoughts were coursing through my brain.

If I did force him to leave, I imagined how he'd describe it to mutual friends the following morning: 'The silly cow threw me out. I thought she was one of the boys and instead she got all jumpy and told me to piss off. As if I'd be interested in that silly, fat bitch.' Those words were so vivid in my mind that I could hear his voice saying them. I couldn't bear the thought of him actually saying that to anyone at all, let alone anyone I knew. Since Kal, I hadn't had a proper relationship with a man. I'd had a brief fling with an old friend from Blackburn, but actors didn't interest me and I was terrified of having a relationship with a stranger in case they sold the story to a tabloid: 'I bedded the fat bird from *Hollyoaks*.'

'It's too late for me to go back to my hotel now. I'm going to have to get in next to you,' he said casually. He could see that I looked horrified. 'Don't be stupid,' he said. 'I'm not gonna try anything.'

I so badly wanted to say to him, 'Get out, get out,' but I just couldn't. My self-esteem was in my boots and my fear of being ostracised, of no longer being one of the boys, stopped me. I had shared my bed with a boy on a purely platonic basis so many times that in general terms it really wasn't a problem for me, but this was different. I felt sick with fear.

He climbed into my bed. At first he just lay there but after a couple of minutes, he rolled onto his front. Then within seconds he was up on his knees and suddenly he had managed to straddle me. He fumbled around in his cheap pants and pulled out what little he found. I was still paralysed and couldn't believe that this was really happening to me. He was trying to get his hand down my pyjama bottoms and was shoving his tongue into my mouth. I had never realised how strong somebody's tongue could be. He was physically smaller than me, but seemed to have this hidden strength. I did try to push him off me, but every time I nearly managed it he would reposition himself to maintain his dominance.

Eventually I managed to speak. It was the only power I had left. 'Please stop. Please, I don't want to. Please.'

He persisted.

'No. NO.' As my voice started to rise, he stopped for a moment, but only a moment.

'Come on, I know you want it.'

At this point I was convinced he was going to rape me and it was inconceivable. I wasn't strong enough to get him off me – my fate was sealed. Then suddenly something switched inside my head, some would say insanity, others self-preservation.

'Please stop, please. I'll give you a blow job if you stop.'

He looked at me for a second but then he continued to tug at the top of my pyjamas. I was by this point very distressed but managed to pull myself together. Very calmly, I said, 'I promise I will give you a blow job if you stop,' and then he leapt into position, grabbing the back of my head and pushing it down. Moments later he relieved himself.

I lay there frozen and distraught for the next four hours in fear that any movement I made would rouse him and that he might still have the urge. Instead he slept like a baby. He woke early and scurried out at about 6 a.m.

I pretended to be asleep when he left, although I'd been sobbing throughout the night. My pillow was sodden with tears. When he left, I sighed heavily with relief. As I took a sharp breath in, I inhaled a mouthful of salty tears from the cotton pillowcase and nearly choked.

I shot out of bed and got dressed. The hotel was in the centre of Manchester and Suranne, or Sarah as I knew her, was filming at Granada, so I ran over there. Fortunately the security guard knew me so allowed me straight up to the *Corrie* green room. I called and left a message on her voicemail en route. She was still listening to the message when I turned up at the door, tear-stained.

As soon as I saw her, I started to cry again. She ushered me into the kitchen, where I poured out everything that had happened.

'Oh, my God, Mikyla, he practically raped you. You can't *not* tell anyone.'

'I have to keep it quiet, Sarah, I just can't tell anyone. You know how it is. The boys will take his side. They'll never understand why I did what I did. Even I don't understand it. It's all too complicated. I wish I could just erase it from my memory. If I tell people, it will follow me around for ever. I just can't do it.'

She hugged me and tried to soothe me, and in the end I went back to the hotel. I stood in the shower and scrubbed and scrubbed at myself.

While I stood in the shower, I could hear my phone ringing over and over again. I knew it would be him. When I eventually got out, I picked up the phone and said, 'Hello,' very coldly.

'What are you going to do about it?' he said, sounding panicked. I knew he was worried that I was going to tell our mutual friend, or even the police, what he had done.

'I haven't decided what I'm going to do yet,' I said icily. 'Now stop calling me. I hope I never have to hear your voice again.'

I put the phone down and sobbed and sobbed. Stupidly, I suppose, I never did report it to the police or tell our mutual friend the unvarnished truth about what happened that night. I was left feeling traumatised and violated, and mixed in with those emotions was a disgust with myself that I hadn't felt I was worthy enough to banish this revolting man from my hotel room. Instead I let him attack me. The idea of that man, or indeed any unwanted man, forcing me to engage in the ultimate intimacy was unthinkable. I couldn't remember a time when I had felt so low.

Although I was very confident in many areas of my life, men were a blind spot where I was unable to afford myself the respect I deserved. I knew that I undervalued myself, but didn't know how to fix it.

One thing I learnt from the experience was never again to allow drugs or alcohol to leave me feeling so alone and exposed.

18

Leaving the Door Open

17 stone 6 pounds

On the top floor of the *Hollyoaks* studios, where the important executives sat in their plush offices, there was a corridor lined with framed magazine covers of cast members. The various slim and gorgeous-looking creatures reclined in scanty underwear, beaming into the camera. For most of the time that I worked at *Hollyoaks* my attitude was positive. I didn't beat myself up about not looking like a size-10 model, I didn't envy those who looked that way or feel inadequate because I was large. I was grateful to have been given the opportunity to be on the show and was determined to be professional and show off my acting ability as far as I could.

The row of magazine covers did rankle, though, and did make me feel like a second-class citizen amongst cast members. I yearned to get on to the cover of a magazine – any magazine – and join the ranks of those immortalised in *FHM*, *Maxim* and the rest.

I did appear on the cover of a property magazine with a couple of other cast members – it was a lovely photo of all of us, and I hoped that at long last my picture would be hung on the top corridor alongside everyone else's. But the decision-makers refused to allow it because it was a free magazine. I was gutted.

Another low point was the shooting of the annual *Hollyoaks* calendar. While many of the Barbie dolls were more than happy to strip down to their skimpiest bikinis and show off their impeccable figures, the whole experience was mortifying for me. The calendar was a vital part of the *Hollyoaks* publicity machine, selling around 100,000 copies. The first year I was at *Hollyoaks* they had a mixed calendar involving the top five boys and girls; in the second year, however, they had separate calendars for boys and girls that involved all permanent cast members, which now included me. I had heard no mention of me going in the calendar at all, until I went into the publicity department and the shoot dates were the topic of conversation.

I rarely had cause to go in there because I rarely did publicity. I can count on the fingers of one hand the number of interviews they put me forward for. Mine wasn't the image they wanted to portray, and the editors of *FHM* and *Maxim* certainly weren't keen for me to grace their pages. This was one area of the soap circus where I always felt second class and surplus to requirements.

There were several of the usual suspects hovering around in publicity, making their routine daily visit to ensure they were at the forefront of the press officers' minds when juicy requests came in for front covers and the like. I did join the conversation about the calendar just so I could throw in the odd sarcastic comment. I had no desire to be a part of it – I didn't want to be like them, but I did feel uncomfortable having the obvious physical differences between us highlighted in this way.

My cynical comments about the calendar often went over the heads of the PR team but amused me immensely. No reference was made to me being involved until I received a call four hours later.

'Mikyla, do you want to be in the calendar?'

'No thank you,' I said without hesitation, and the conversation ended there.

The next day I received a call from Jo Hallows's office and was summoned upstairs. This would have filled some people with dread, but I was able to speak freely to Jo and knew she was fair so was happy to go and see her.

'What's all this nonsense about you not doing the calendar?' she asked without even so much as a hello. She did put me a little on the back foot, but I believed I was morally right.

'I don't want to do it. I'm an actress, not a model, and besides, the people buying that calendar don't want to see me any more than I want to be in the stupid thing.'

She looked me straight in the eye. Despite her petite stature, there was nothing diminutive about Jo's presence. If she fixed you with a stare, you knew about it.

'You're wrong, Mikyla, very wrong. Your absence from that calendar would speak volumes in a very negative way. It would imply you are less attractive or desirable than the other girls and not worthy of a place. You should celebrate the way you look and I can assure you there are plenty of people who would be more than happy to look at a picture of you.'

'But—'

'Nobody's asking you to wear a bikini. We'll find something you are comfortable in.'

'But—'

'Before you offer any more objections, I can tell you I'm not interested in hearing them. You're going to appear in that calendar. End of.'

So that was that. Into the calendar I went. I know she was right, but it didn't make the physical process any easier.

The other actresses had been preparing themselves for the shoot with extended sunbed sessions. I knew that I never, ever wanted to be seen in a bikini and had to plan the most tasteful possible cover-up. It wasn't only hard for me but also for any other girl who didn't look like a perfect pin-up, even if she was considered very attractive compared with the general population.

When the calendar was shot that second year at *Hollyoaks*, we were flown to Majorca and accommodated in two villas – one was for the crew and the other for the girls. The crew got the attractive villa, while we got the ugly concrete one. There was an old-fashioned picture of Jesus on the stairs. I'm not religious, but every time I gazed at that picture I felt like a sinner.

I decided to take the picture down while we were in residence and rehung it when we left. After much draping of black negligees, it was decided to only do a head and shoulders shot of me. I was very happy to have my body out of the picture. While I had become an expert at shrugging off comments about my size, it didn't mean that moments of juxtaposition with *Hollyoaks*'s classic calendar girls weren't terribly painful for me.

Once the decision had been taken to do a headshot of me, I wondered why I had had to travel all the way to Majorca when I could have stayed on the *Hollyoaks* set in Liverpool. Instead I was flown out to the middle of nowhere in the baking-hot sun to sit like a vampire in the shade and watch ten blondes and a brunette recline in the sun. They took great interest in each other's Polaroid shots and offered suggestions about how to improve their already goddess-like appearances. This was torture for me, but I couldn't escape. There was no TV and nowhere to walk to. I just had to sit and listen to lots of superficial rubbish. To give me that holiday look, the make-up artist decided to apply fake tan. An eerie orange glow on a woman with very white freckled skin isn't a look I'm in favour of, but pale and interesting wasn't the remit so we did the best we could.

When I saw the final calendar, I wasn't particularly pleased with the result. It was obvious why everyone else had their whole body on show while only my head and shoulders were visible. I gritted my teeth when I looked at the finished calendar. I knew Jo had been right to insist that I took part, but it didn't make looking at the final product any more comfortable for me.

During my time at *Hollyoaks* I frequently managed to put my foot in it. I sometimes speak without thinking. That can be refreshing, particularly in the showbiz world, which is often very false and sycophantic. But there were times when I wished I could have caught my words and stuffed them back into my clumsy mouth.

One cringe-worthy moment that still makes me giggle now involved Gemma Atkinson when she first joined the show aged fifteen to play Lisa Hunter in the newly established Hunter family. Due to her age, Gemma's mum, Sandra, had to attend the studio and act as a chaperone to Gemma, so I had often chatted to her and offered advice regarding an agent and guidelines on the fee percentage they should expect to pay. Gemma has now developed into a stunning young woman and even at the tender age of fifteen projected an incredible amount of sex appeal. She was supposed to be a schoolgirl harbouring a dark family secret, while appearing very pure and innocent. You can imagine my confusion when I walked into the green room to find Gemma kitted out in a school uniform that you would expect to see in an Ann Summers catalogue. As I sat down and studied this costume more closely, I was alarmed at the shortness of the grey school skirt that just about grazed her knickerline and the white shirt that stretched across her sizeable bust, creating a prominent cleavage. I decided I should step in and offer my advice on this matter and encourage her mother to complain about her daughter being given such an indecent costume.

'Sandra, I'm sorry but that uniform is not acceptable. There are plenty of older girls that are more than happy to flash some thigh or accentuate their bust to satisfy the army of men who watch this show just to gawp at the women. Go to wardrobe and tell them you are not prepared to let them exploit your daughter. Do they realise she is only fifteen?'

Sandra looked at me for a moment and smiled. Then she said, 'I agree it's not acceptable. The only trouble is, Mikyla, Gemma hasn't got changed yet. That's her own school uniform!'

I was momentarily lost for words, but seconds later we all erupted into howls of laughter. I know this moment won me a place in Sandra's heart. From then on she trusted me to watch out for Gemma in the crazy world of soaps. I would often have Gemma pass the phone to my ear at 3 a.m. and I'd hear a sleepy Sandra say, 'Is Gemma there with you, Mikyla?' and a simple yes (which was about all I could usually manage at that time of night) would put her mind at rest. I looked upon Gemma as a little sister and was extremely protective towards her. I was wary of her ending up in a hotel room like I did taking cocaine just because it was offered. My efforts paid off and Gemma has negotiated her way around the usual temptations and grown into a smart young girl who I am incredibly proud of.

One year on my birthday, I texted various friends along with members of the cast and crew to say I was going to Jalon's to celebrate my birthday and asking if anyone fancied coming along. Twenty-three people came, along with my mum, my dad and my auntie Barbara, who was an actress and loved being surrounded by actor types.

That evening in the restaurant was the first time ever that my dad had stepped into my world and was surrounded by people whom I knew well and accepted me for all my flaws. My dad ended up sitting with Ben Hull, who was a much-loved friend.

I had discussed with Ben at length my strange relationship with my parents. I knew he would be waxing lyrical about how much fun I was and how well I was doing. I didn't pay too much attention, but I could see my dad looked like a fish out of water. He seemed awkward, but chatted away and tried to appear interested. For the first time in my life I wasn't concerned about what he would say – I was quite simply indifferent. I reasoned if he was being nice, then great and even if he was being false or if he was mean, I knew there were more than enough people to defend my honour and he would only look silly.

I can't describe how relieved I felt. I had spent my entire life feeling like I wasn't good enough or that I should have been a boy or that I was an inconvenience, and suddenly I felt fine. It was like a grey cloud had been lifted and I was at last free of these inadequate feelings and the sense of being in the way.

I had a dream job, and a group of fabulous friends new and old. Not to mention that by this stage, I had taken another step and bought my own house and had a BMW on the drive. Meanwhile my dad had exactly what he wanted: my mum all to himself. Then I started to think how sad I was for him that parenthood hadn't been the joy it is for so many and that in turn made his pride in my success bittersweet. Then my attention was distracted by the arrival of my birthday cake. John, the owner, had been out and bought the biggest cake you've ever seen and everybody started singing. Several vodkas later I was stood up watching my friend Danny who was playing the in-house piano. (Yes, that's right – the Soap Awards fake boyfriend is not only good-looking but can sing *and* play the piano.) He sang a couple of Take That songs to huge applause. I looked around the room feeling a real sense of happiness in a way I never had before. Then I spotted my dad, who, not being a fan of loud music, had sloped off. I don't know what possessed me to do this, but I wandered up behind him and put my arms round him from behind.

'All right, love?' he said in a warm, upbeat way.

'Yeah, I'm all right. I hope you've had a good time. I love it here and I wish you could enjoy it as much as I do. These people know me and love me, and what's more they tell me they love me. It makes me incredibly sad that you don't tell me you love me.'

He continued looking straight ahead but rubbed my arm, which was still securely wrapped round him, and spoke quietly. 'My dad didn't tell me either, so it doesn't come easily.'

Being drunk, I barely drew breath before retaliating. 'That's not a good enough excuse. You don't tell me, but I'm damn sure that when I have kids they will know how much I love them and not just because I tell them so but because of the way I behave and how interested I'll be in everything they do or say. I've not had that. I constantly question whether you love me.'

'I do love you, but I just don't say it.'

I paused for a moment. 'I know you do, but I need to know you like me as well and that you enjoy being around me, just like all these people here tonight. I no longer need your approval or care about whether you disagree with things I do or say, but I would like you to get to know me better and want to spend time with me. I'm actually a pretty cool girl who is popular because I would do anything for anybody, and I want you to see that in me.' I suddenly felt a wet drop on my arm, and realising what it was, my own voice started to wobble. I squeezed him tightly and continued: 'From now on I'm not going to come over to Blackburn and plonk myself in front of the TV with you. That's too easy. If you want to see me, then you have got to make the effort. My door will be wide open.'

I hurriedly wiped my eyes and then returned to the party, leaving my dad staring out of the window of the crowded restaurant. Shortly after that my mum and auntie left, along with my very quiet dad.

My mum rang me first thing the next morning with no thought for my killer hangover. 'What did you say to your dad?'

Weirdly I didn't feel comfortable telling her. It was between me and him, and for the first time she wasn't having to mediate or edit what had been said by the other as she so often did. I felt vindicated and relieved to have said my piece. I asked my mum what my dad had said to her.

'Nothing, not a word. He was just silent the whole way home and went straight to bed.'

I was sure that my words had sunk in and that maybe things could change. I'd often imagined that that moment would have to wait until one of us was on our death bed. I was over the moon that it hadn't taken that long for me to say what I desperately needed to say to my dad. All in all, that evening was one of the happiest in my life.

19
Camilla Parker-Bowles and Me

18 stone

If three magic ingredients are placed together – me, Sarah (Suranne) Jones and alcohol – the outcome will always be mischief. The night before we went to Prince Charles's charity polo match was no exception.

An anonymous admirer had sent Sarah a pay-as-you-go mobile phone with a message asking her to call the number saved in the memory after she'd made herself a potent cocktail containing the bottles of champagne, Angostura bitters and brandy that he had sent her. The message said, 'I promise you once you have drunk this cocktail, you will pick up this phone and dial the only number stored in it.'

We made up the cocktail, which was incredibly potent, and rang the number, but Sarah declined his invitation to take her out for dinner. It was 4 a.m. when the two of us crawled into bed extremely drunk.

A car was due to collect us at some unearthly hour like 8 a.m. to go to the polo match. When the car arrived, we were both fast asleep. We mumbled some excuse to the driver, who we knew wouldn't have been expecting a pair of actors to be ready on time. Twenty minutes later we'd thrown on some clothes we hoped would be suitable for a polo match and were clutching our make-up bags. Sarah wore a yellow and white dress, and I put on a red top with a low, scalloped neck and a long, thick, black skirt that hugged my curves. We reasoned that we'd have plenty of time to tart ourselves up and conceal the dark, hungover circles under our eyes while we were in the car.

When we arrived, we instantly downed the champagne and Pimm's being offered to us by polite waiters carrying silver trays.

'Hair of the dog is the only way,' I said to Sarah, gulping back mine.

It was a beautiful day. The sun was shining, and an exquisitely decorated marquee had been laid on for the lunch we were going to eat before the polo match began. Jamie Oliver was doing the catering.

Both Suranne's and my eyes were on stalks when we spotted John Travolta, a huge hero for both of us, seated next to Joan Rivers, a wonderful, hilarious woman who describes things exactly as she sees them. I had loved *Grease* so much when I was growing up that I had worn out my video of it from constantly replaying the final part. 'Tell me about it, Stud.'

When we sat down for lunch, Sarah and I sat next to Helen Worth, who plays Gail Platt on *Coronation Street*. She had just been to Elton John's tiara ball and regaled us with stories about the celebrities who were there.

We were served something that we thought might be

guinea fowl – not a food that any of us were too familiar with.

Emboldened by several glasses of champagne and Pimm's, I said cheerily, 'Oh, well, there's only one way to find out,' and rammed my fork into the flesh. It was indeed guinea fowl and copious amounts of guinea-fowl fat splattered all over my lovely red top.

'Oh, dear,' said Helen. 'There's no point sponging fat off, it'll just make it worse. You better leave it as it is.'

'Oh, no,' I griped. 'I can't go up and say hello to John Travolta splattered in guinea-fowl fat.'

Then the polo match commenced. We were seated next to a pleasant woman called Lady Sarah Apsley. She had never watched *Hollyoaks* or indeed anything on Channel 4 but was a huge fan of *Coronation Street*. She kept on referring to her husband as 'Lord Apsley', and in my inebriated state this made me giggle. I'd never heard of anyone referring to their husband as Lord anyone before.

In the end, perplexed by my giggling, she said, 'Are you all right?'

'Oh, yes, I'm fine,' I replied. 'I just find it funny that you refer to your husband as Lord Apsley rather than by his Christian name.'

She looked surprised. 'But that is his name.' She continued to chat away and I continued to giggle every time she said 'Lord Apsley', until eventually she turned to me and very politely yet absent-mindedly said, 'What is it about Lord Apsley's name that amuses you so?'

'Doesn't he have a Christian name?' I asked.

'Yes, he does.' She paused and with a devilish twinkle in her eye, said, 'It's Geoffrey.'

Now it was her turn to burst out laughing, leaving me quite confused as to what she now found so amusing. 'Not really,' she said eventually. 'But how funny would that be?'

Sarah and I threw each other wide-eyed looks and smiled exaggeratedly to cover our bewilderment. This wasn't the working class humour we were familiar with – too upper-class for two scallys.

Changing the subject, Lady Apsley said, 'Have you met the prince before?'

'Oh, yes, Suranne and I are very lucky. We met him at the Children of Courage Awards.'

She nodded and smiled. 'And have you met Camilla?'

Both of us shook our heads. Then I stood there with a full glass of champagne in my hand, in my guinea fowl-splattered top, while Camilla came over and beamed at us.

Because of the media reporting and the Princess Diana situation, I had a very negative image of Camilla, but in the flesh she was smiley and charming and appeared to be a very nice, warm, normal woman, not at all the gargoyle of popular mythology. The conversation focused on Suranne and her role in *Coronation Street*, but Sarah tried to bring me into the conversation.

'My friend's also a soap actress,' she began.

'Yes,' said Lady Apsley. 'This is Suranne's friend Michelle, who's in something on Channel 4.'

I can't pretend this didn't bother me, just as it does when people mistake me for Jennie McAlpine, who plays Fiz on

Coronation Street. As the conversation continued to focus on Suranne, the group almost had its back to me. I decided this wasn't how it was going to work – perhaps I got a touch of the green-eyed monster.

I shakily switched my glass of champagne from my right hand to my left and touched Camilla's arm with my right hand.

''Ere,' I confided, 'we wanna know how come you got to sit next to John Travolta.'

She looked at me in amazement. This was obviously not a question that anyone else at the polo match had asked her.

'Is it because you know the govern'r?'

Camilla tried to smile politely and then with the alacrity of a greyhound she was off. Sarah gave me a dirty look, which said silently, 'You twat.' I carried on drunkenly sipping my champagne.

Although Sarah was much less drunk than I was, I could see that she was giggling behind her annoyance. The whole thing was like a scene from car-crash TV.

As we stood people-watching, the word went round that John Travolta was leaving.

'I've got to say something to him,' I said to Sarah, and strode purposefully in his direction.

I marched up to him and shook his hand. 'Look at you, with your dimples and your big blue eyes,' I slurred.

Never before or since has anyone snatched their hand out of mine so speedily. Sarah was mortified.

'I must go to the loo,' I said, sighing as I watched John Travolta hurry off.

There were upmarket temporary toilets in the grounds,

and after trying to sober up by splashing water on my face, I felt a little better.

'I'm all right now,' I called out to Suranne. 'I've washed my face and I'm feeling much better.' Then I toppled over and fell backwards into the toilet cubicle I'd just emerged from.

'Mikyla, enough, go and sit in the car until it's time to go,' said Suranne.

It made a refreshing change as I'm normally Captain Sensible even after a couple of bottles of whatever's on the menu.

I never did get invited to Prince Charles's polo match again. Oops.

I did meet Tony Blair, though, when he came with Cherie to visit the set of *Hollyoaks*. The soap's creator, Phil Redmond, was a staunch Labour supporter. I'm not a person who holds strong political views, but I had been impressed by Tony Blair's performance after the death of Princess Diana.

As we lined up to meet Tony and Cherie, I stood between the actors Jimmy McKenna, who played Jack Osbourne, and Paul Byatt, who played Mick Dixon in Brookside. Jimmy was dressed casually in an open-necked polo shirt. He was very excited about meeting Tony Blair and was perspiring on his forehead. He complimented Mr Blair on his premiership. Then the prime minister moved on to shake hands with me, and as he did I heard Paul saying from my right, 'Look at Jimmy, he's sweating like a rapist.'

I just stood there clutching the prime minister's hand, open-mouthed. Blair didn't know quite how to take that remark and moved swiftly on, flashing his trademark smile. Paul was pure Scouser. His bluntness around the prime minister summed up everything I loved about Liverpool and its inhabitants.

20
'People Die From That'

17 stone 7 pounds

Having been in *Hollyoaks* for well over three years I felt very at home there. I hadn't had a major storyline for a while, but everything seemed to be running smoothly. The cast members and the crew had become my extended family, and I spent a lot of days in between filming cracking jokes and laughing at people's quips. I had no sense at all of what was about to hit me, when the phone rang.

It was one of the casting assistants. She told me I needed to go to the office to sign my new contract. This was a routine annual event that took place about four or five months before current contracts expired in order for storylines to advance, so I thought nothing of it.

'Sure, I'll pop along soon,' I said.

'Oh, and by the way,' she said airily, 'your new contract is only for six months.'

I couldn't believe what I was hearing. I'd had a few conversations with some of the production team about my readiness to go, but this wasn't how I expected it to happen. I certainly didn't expect to hear this life-changing news in such a blasé fashion.

'Six months? Are you sure?' I hoped she'd made a mistake.

'Yes, I'm sure. This has come straight from Jo Hallows. They only need you for six months.'

I'd been lulled into a false sense of security on the show, even though I wasn't part of a *Hollyoaks* family, who could have acted as a buffer against dismissal. I had thought that the relationships I had built and the hard work I had done entitled me to a little more than having this enormous bombshell dropped over the phone.

I put down the phone and immediately called Jo Hallows's office.

'I need to see Jo. Is she around?' I asked.

Her secretary, Lisa, could tell something was wrong as I wasn't my usual chatty self. I sounded cold and businesslike and was desperately trying to hold things together. 'Is everything all right, Miky?' she asked in her warm Scouse accent.

'Not really. Apparently I'm only getting a six-month contract and the first I heard of it was from casting two minutes ago.'

Jo was available later that day, but I was on set filming until late. I was constantly checking my watch hoping that she hadn't gone home. I hadn't told anybody on set yet because I was too upset. The only person who knew was Nick Pickard, who plays Tony, and I had burst into tears as I told him. I can't explain how heartbreaking it was. He and I had so many fun memories of late nights listening to Stevie Wonder and Frank Sinatra. We'd been on holiday together; I'd even spent Christmas Day with his fantastic family. I couldn't believe all this was going be taken away from me.

For him, it was strange because I was one of the last of his old schoolmates. 'The party crew' were a dying breed. He had been here so many times before, having to say goodbye to one of his best pals.

It was 7.30 p.m. by the time I got off set. I immediately called Jo on her mobile.

'Hi, Miky. I'm still here. Come on up,' she said.

She was sitting in the now-deserted open-plan office all packed up and ready to walk out the door and was waiting patiently for me. Before I could speak she jumped straight in and apologised: 'I'm sorry – you weren't supposed to find out like that. The decision was only made late last night, and it's nine months, not six. This way you'll be finishing just before the summer so will have more chance of finding something else.'

At that point I was still unsure of whether to sign, but the reality was, I would need to stay for financial stability, so I reluctantly agreed on the basis that my character would get a positive leaving story. Jo was true to her word, and I was busy for the remainder of my time there.

Although I now lived in Liverpool, I went back to Blackburn fairly regularly. Sam had moved to France, and Jay was still away in the army, but I saw the other members of the family. I adored Cameron and Preshella, the two children Ella had with Precious, and tried to see them whenever I could. Cameron looks like Ella and laughs like her – throwing his whole head and body back. He's a real bundle of joy and brought Ella enormous happiness. Like my mum, she had always adored babies.

Ella's health seemed to be stable although as ever quite fragile. Then suddenly, out of the blue, she was diagnosed with bowel cancer. The consultant was very upbeat about her chances of beating it, and I had complete faith in him. I wasn't one of those people who went hysterical at the mention of the word 'cancer'. I thought of all Ella's previous health problems and how she had come through them and was sure that in the same way that she'd dealt with her ulcerative colitis and her asthma she'd deal with bowel cancer.

I cuddled her after the diagnosis and said, 'We'll get through this, Ella, we will.'

She nodded. Like me, she seemed positive about the prognosis and said she wanted to start the treatment as soon as possible.

During the next few months I worked at a relentless pace. As Jo had promised, I wasn't going to go out of *Hollyoaks* with a whimper. But every spare moment I had I spent with Ella and was constantly going from Liverpool to Blackburn to visit her.

She underwent major surgery to remove the cancer, and afterwards we all had different roles to play in her life. I was chief buyer of beautiful flowers and appetising food, which I hoped would tempt her to eat. If she had requested quail's eggs and caviar, I would have obliged if only to get her to eat something and put a smile on her face.

The flowers became a running joke. I once showed up empty-handed.

'No flowers?' she asked cheekily.

'No, I'm sure somebody will bring some,' I said. I had already considered getting a weekend job in order to fund her floral requirements.

'Nobody else brings them now – you scared them off,' she said.

Apparently other people would arrive with service-station offerings of daffodils or carnations, cringe when they saw my splendid offering and never bother again.

Jay fulfilled a different role. He made Ella laugh. He sat by her bedside for hours on end holding her hand. There wasn't an enormous amount to laugh about as she got sicker and sicker, but the worse things got, the more she needed to be able to laugh.

Ella's husband, Precious, was illiterate and couldn't sign forms, do the household paperwork or even follow a shopping list, so this left him rather redundant. He was, however, very capable around the house, and where domestic chores were concerned, he excelled.

My sister Sam came over from France to help. She and my mum ferried Ella back and forth from her hospital appointments as I was often at work. One day she had a scan followed by an appointment to discuss the results and find out whether the cancer had spread.

The appointment was in the forefront of my mind, and my mum had agreed to keep me posted. I was in Liverpool city centre dressed as a nun for my *Hollyoaks* hen night – Chloe had got back together with Kristian's character and was marrying him. I was filming with Elize du Toit, who played Izzy. She and I had a strained relationship at the best of times, so I wasn't in the greatest of moods. Then I received a text from my mum. I was delighted, assuming it must be positive news or she wouldn't be communicating via text. I opened the text and my face dropped. I looked up at the sky and did quite literally feel as if my world was falling in. The cast and crew looked the same as they had a few moments ago, but something in me had changed for ever. I felt sick and dizzy. At that moment I didn't want to go on, not just with the scene but with anything.

My mum's text read baldly, 'It's in the liver.'

I slumped into the chair I was standing over. The assistant director rushed to me and asked if I was OK.

I had gone into shock and couldn't think of anything diplomatic to say. I blurted out, 'My sister's got cancer of the liver.'

Everybody went silent, until someone said, 'Oh, my God, people die from that!'

'Thanks for that.' I grimaced. 'I know people die from it.' Tears started to roll down my cheeks.

That was the first moment I actually acknowledged that Ella might die. She was my big sister, one of my best friends, Rosco, Cameron and Preshella's mummy and my mum's daughter. How would my mum take it? It's not natural for a parent to see their child die.

As if the day wasn't bad enough, the location camera stopped working and we had to wait for a new one to be delivered. I decided I needed a drink. By the time the camera arrived I was drunk, which wasn't the end of the world as I was supposed to be in exactly that state for the scene. It was one of those moments of method acting.

Ella's initial surgery was to remove her bowel and re-place it with a colostomy bag. This is a man-made bowel constructed out of rubbery plastic that sits on the exterior of the body and needs to be emptied on a regular basis. Once that horrible bag was attached, I think she lost the will to live. She needed a course of chemotherapy to shrink the liver cancer and then had to be operated on again. Like so many people, she contracted MRSA, which dragged her down hugely. Ella was a woman who had always chatted about her home, her kids and what she'd seen on TV. When she was diagnosed with cancer, she didn't much feel like small talk any more and became very quiet. She rarely talked about her death, but when she lay stricken with the MRSA, she said, 'I don't think this is going to have a happy ending.'

Once she recovered from the MRSA, she needed a cannula in her hand for chemotherapy treatment. She refused to go, weary of being prodded and poked. I was in Liverpool working on *Hollyoaks* and I screamed down the phone to my mum that somehow she had to get Ella to hospital for that treatment.

'If she doesn't have that cannula put in, she can't have the chemo and she *will* die, so I don't care how much she doesn't want it, she's going.'

They did manage to get her to the hospital and had the cannula inserted into her weak grey hand, but three days later, when the time came for her first bout of chemotherapy, she just didn't have the strength for it. It became clear we had little time left.

Precious, Sam and I stayed at the hospital with other members of the family dropping in. It all seemed to happen so quickly, and there were a million things I wanted to say to her but none of them seemed appropriate. I'd always looked to her to set the tone, but she was already so far away from the sister I knew and loved.

Ella was our big sister. She got on better with each of us than any of us did with each other and soothed us back on to speaking terms whenever we fell out. She never thought the worst of anybody and went through life in a placid, peaceable way, harming no one and exercising quiet diplomacy that acted as a balm in our volatile family. I couldn't believe that this was it.

There were lots of practical things to be done, and it fell upon Jay and me to do them. She hadn't made a will and so he had to make a frantic dash to WH Smith to buy a DIY one. Ella was lying in her hospital bed in agony by this time, but we asked the nurse to hold off from giving her a higher dose of morphine so that she could remain 'of sound mind' until she had signed her will and said goodbye to her two young children.

I went to collect Preshella and Cameron, who were ready for school. They didn't really understand that their mum was close to death and bounced into her hospital room.

Cameron spied a yoghurt on top of Ella's locker, which we'd tried and failed to tempt Ella to eat. 'Mum, can I have that yoghurt?' said Cameron breezily. Ella was too exhausted to speak, but nodded weakly.

Jay had spoken to them outside Ella's room and explained that their mum was very poorly and that it would make her happy to hear them tell her they loved her. Cameron nodded, but Shella wasn't going to oblige. It was as if, instinctively, she knew that that meant it was the end.

Cameron said, 'I love you, Mummy. Bye-bye.' He was keen to get to school.

Forcing myself not to cry in front of the children, I drove them to school.

I was greeted at the school gates by a panicked-looking head teacher. I stepped out of the car and he said quietly and urgently, 'Do the children know their mum's going to die?'

I shook my head. We'd decided this would distress them and that Jay should tell them once she had gone, as neither I nor Precious was brave enough.

'Well, all the other children at the school do because your neighbour's child has told them, so Cameron and Shella simply can't come into school today.'

Cameron was dying to go into school and kicked up an enormous fuss about it. 'Why? Why? You promised we could go to school. You lied!'

It was unbearable. I wanted to scream, but I couldn't explain to them that in a few short hours they wouldn't have a mummy and that school wasn't important right now. Somehow I managed to persuade them to leave school and took them to a neighbour's house until my auntie could collect them. I promised I'd return soon and raced back to the hospital. Ella had signed her will and had been given a strong dose of morphine, which sent her into a deep daze. The whole family sat around her bed, with Sam and my mum willing her to keep on breathing. I prayed that she'd stop breathing as soon as possible because I couldn't bear for her pain to go on any longer.

She took her last breath around 11.45 a.m. on 9 October. Precious wailed as she left us, which is traditional in St Lucia. It upset my mum immensely because she felt it wasn't very dignified, but he was Ella's husband so what could we say.

My auntie Helen is a Macmillan nurse. She and I laid Ella out. We tenderly gave her a bed bath, and I plaited her hair before changing her into a fresh nightie and removing the colostomy bag she despised so much.

I had a peculiar feeling that while I was doing those things for her she was still with us. I could almost hear her thinking, When you leave the room, I'll go and see what's happening up there on the other side.

I don't think there are many people in my life I could do that for. It would freak me out too much, but it really did seem like the right thing to do for my beloved sister.

She had never been a religious person, but at the age of nineteen she had had a very bad asthma attack and her heart had stopped beating. She was brought back with a shot of adrenaline but later told us that she'd travelled down a white tunnel and had seen a man with a white beard wearing a white suit looking like someone out of the Bee Gees. She knew she wasn't ready to go there and came back to us. After that she always said she didn't fear death. 'When the time comes, I know I'll be all right. I know there's a place for me to go,' she told us.

In the days after Ella's death, Rosco did a lot of crying. My mum was emotional but got on with doing the things she had to do to prepare for the funeral. Thankfully my dad kept quiet. I went into my florist in Liverpool and told her that we wanted something lovely and bright from the children. The children had been in with me once when Ella was ill and had told the florist that there were two things their mum loved: pretty flowers and sucking on boiled sweets. The florist had remembered and surpassed herself with the arrangement she made for us. She had produced beautiful bouquets of parrot tulips, sunflowers, roses and fragrant freesias. The flowers were so bright and optimistic, and as a final, thoughtful touch the florist had remembered Shella's comment and threaded boiled sweets and little lollipops in amongst the flowers.

I had bought Shella a red top and black skirt for the funeral. Precious's mother had travelled from St Lucia. When she saw Shella in the outfit about an hour before the funeral service was due to begin, she threw up her hands in horror and started screaming as if someone else had died.

'You can't have the child wearing red for a funeral – it's terrible bad luck. No one would ever wear red to a funeral in St Lucia.'

Judging by her hysteria, the situation was non-negotiable so in a dreamlike state, as if trapped in some sort of black comedy, I raced down to Asda and grabbed several non-red tops for Shella in the hope that they would appease Precious's mum.

We had chosen three songs for the funeral: 'The Wind Beneath My Wings', Heather Small's 'Proud' and her namesake Ella Fitzgerald's 'Every Time We Say Goodbye'.

My mum and Sam had been keen for Ella's children not to go to the funeral, but I had felt very strongly that they should be there so that they could say goodbye to their mum. I knew that Precious would be open to suggestions about whether the children should go or not, and had decided that I must get to him before my mum and Sam did. I had raced round to Ella's house where he was staying and begged him to allow them to go to the funeral. He had agreed. My mum was furious at the time, but I was absolutely convinced that I'd done the right thing and I now know my mum agrees.

At the funeral Rosco was seated in between Jay and me. Sam was hanging off my mum's arm sobbing uncontrollably. Somehow Shella ended up sitting next to Sam and didn't really understand how funerals worked.

'Auntie Sam, who's in that box?' she said in a loud voice, pointing to the coffin.

Sam became hysterical, but Jay, Rosco and I actually chuckled. The congregation must have thought we'd gone mad.

Somehow we got through the funeral service. The music we'd chosen was interspersed with our sad, funny and touching Ella stories. I volunteered to do the eulogy and tried desperately to separate myself and treat it like a performance to prevent me from falling apart and letting Ella down.

There were so many wonderful things that simply had to be said. I remembered the time I wrote off a Ford Fiesta that I'd saved and saved for. I'd been out with my dad, who was giving me a driving lesson. I couldn't brake in time and collided with another car. Fortunately nobody was hurt, but the car was only fit for the scrap yard. I was heartbroken, until Ella turned up with a bunch of flowers and a copy of *Autotrader*. By the end of the same day I had another Fiesta and a two-year plan to repay her – God, I loved her.

The crematorium was bursting at the seams, and I'd promised the children that if they behaved throughout the service they could eat the sweets from the bouquets at the end. They did behave and, oblivious to the devastation around them, were more than ready to collect their reward. I thought it was fitting that the sweets were Ella's last little gift to her children. And besides, she never did like to see things go to waste.

21
Jude Law Wasn't Late

18 stone

By the end of June 2004 *Hollyoaks* was over for me, but
Chloe went out on a high. Ironically she landed a better
job than I did when I left the soap – she got a position as
an apprentice DJ on London's Capital Radio. About four
months before my departure from *Hollyoaks*, I decided it
was time to find an agent. I had finally ditched the one
who couldn't get my name right. I wasn't the kind of
person to do lots of research into this. Several of my
friends and ex-co-stars were with a particular agency and
suggested I follow suit, so I did. I met the only female
agent in the team. She was pleasant enough and we
chatted casually about my situation and what I wanted
from the future.

'We'd be delighted to look after you, Mikyla,' she said. It
all seemed a bit too easy. It was a very reputable agency
with lots of high-profile clients. Surely I needed to do more
than just chat politely to be invited into the fold.

'That's great, but please don't take me just because you
haven't got a "fat girl" on your books. Take me because
you believe you can help to mould my career.'

'Absolutely. I assure you, Mikyla, we push our artists a

hundred per cent and totally believe in their ability and talent above anything aesthetic.'

What a great answer, I thought to myself. How lucky I am to have landed such an amazing agent. Maybe life after *Hollyoaks* is going to be bright after all.

The agency sent me along to a photographer to get my head and shoulder portraits done.

'He's expensive, darling, but he's worth it,' breathed my new agent.

I found my way to the man's studio near Sloane Square but not knowing London very well, I was about half an hour late for the appointment.

The studio was stunning, spacious and minimalist. He invited me in and went to fetch some different camera lenses. I looked around. I noticed a magnificent black-and-white portrait of Jude Law in a dinner jacket with a bottle of whisky dangling from his hand.

'Did you see the photograph of Jude Law?' the photographer asked me, when he came back into the studio. He was a small, slight man with wiry grey hair and a strong Eastern European accent. He looked like a mad Russian inventor.

'Yes, it's great. What was he like?' I asked.

'On time,' he said pointedly.

He didn't seem to bear a grudge about my poor time-keeping, though, and proceeded to set up the shoot.

'Do you want to do the make-up?' he said, making a flicking movement near his eye.

'You mean mascara?' I said.

'Yes, yes,' he said.

'OK, then.'

I left him fiddling with his lights and went into the bathroom to put on my make-up. When I returned, he was still fiddling with the lights.

His mobile phone rang and irritably he picked it up. 'Who is this disturbing me when I'm photographing such a beauty?' he muttered to himself before he took the call. 'Yes, yes, I'll call you back. I'm busy right now.' He hung up. 'That was some Appleton girl. Who is that?'

'It's probably one of the singers from the band All Saints,' I said. 'They're very famous.' His response was simply, 'OK, maybe I take her picture.'

He spent a long time photographing me.

'You want to be like you make love to the camera?'

I shook my head.

'OK, you don't like, no problem.'

He continued snapping me and told me he'd send prints through in a couple of weeks.

I left unsure whether he was a total genius or stark-raving mad. When I saw the pictures, I knew it was the first option. These were quite simply the best photographs I'd ever seen of myself. The lighting he used flattered my features and my skin tone perfectly. I was certain that the photographs were a good omen and that my phone would be ringing constantly with offers of work and auditions, thanks to my new agent.

My newfound optimism encouraged me to sell my house in Liverpool and buy a flat in London. I decided on East London. The decision about the 2012 Olympics was pending and I thought it would be a good investment if we won the bid. I didn't know a soul in East London, though. Gary Lucy and his family lived out in Essex. My friends Julie and

Claire Buckfield lived in North London, and my cousin, Kim, and aunt in West London. If we didn't get the Olympics, I was going to end up lonely and poor. Thankfully my gamble paid off.

I had a big *Hollyoaks* leaving party, which happened to fall on the night England lost spectacularly to Portugal in Euro 2004 on 24 June. In any other city this wouldn't have been an issue, but in Liverpool football is religion. Watching Stevie Gerrard and the England boys suffer so unfairly was enough to ruin any party. I was delighted to see so many people make the effort, despite their heavy hearts. One of our lovely camera operators did point out that if it had been anybody apart from me having a party, the room would probably have been empty and that was testament to my popularity, which touched me greatly. I said goodbye to so many people who had helped me through some of my darkest and happiest moments. There had been times I had felt alienated and alone, but they had been more than compensated for by huge amounts of fun.

My move to London went well. My mum and dad had by this time moved to France, but my dad was more than happy to come over and help me move from one end of the country to the other.

Once I was settled and my flatmate Russell had moved in, it was time to get a job. I called my new agent and suggested lunch.

'OK, babe, how about a week on Friday?' I didn't have much choice but to accept this advance booking, but being impatient as I am, I wanted her to say tomorrow.

The day came and she postponed our meeting until the following Thursday. We went for a quiet lunch and chatted about this and that – holidays, music and the like. Often small talk is essential in these situations.

Then I asked the fatal question: 'Is there much work around at the moment?' I expected there would at least be the suggestion of a panto or a general meeting, which is just a sit-down with a casting director. It's speculative and not necessarily for a particular role.

Her response was simple. 'Nothing suitable for you, darling, but be patient.' Then she went back to the office and I paid the bill.

That was the last time I saw her.

I wanted to scream at her, 'Find me a bloody job, any job. I'm going insane.' But instead I agreed to follow her advice and 'be patient'.

Then I was sent to a cattle-market audition for a commercial. The type you see advertised in the paper. I couldn't understand it – why was I not being sent for proper auditions? Programmes were being made, and surely somebody wanted to see me even if only as a favour to my agent.

I started to feel very low and rejected. I couldn't help but wonder as I had before *Hollyoaks* if my appearance was the main thing holding me back.

If it was my size that was preventing me achieving further success, I realised I was in trouble, because I am never going to be a size 10. The reason being, I'm 6 foot tall and have an ample frame to begin with. I'm like an Amazon and I simply enjoy food, maybe too much to work at becoming wafer thin. I really do love eating well; without it my life would be miserable and we shouldn't exist to be miserable. The problem for me is that like anything that makes you happy you need a lot of it if you are unhappy. When my life is going well, I eat a lot, but I'm not a gannet and I don't occupy my mind with what my next meal is going to be. When I'm unhappy, food becomes a means of survival. Instead of thinking about what is wrong in my life, I divert my attention to food.

So began the same downward spiral as before. I began to eat to numb the pain and worry of being overweight. It's a self-fulfilling, lose-lose situation fuelled by pain.

Nearly a year passed with not a single acting job and I was beside myself. If I'd gone to auditions and not got the job, I'd have understood, but instead I wasn't even being seen, so there was no opportunity to prove myself. I would only get a call if they wanted a fat actress to play a character related to being fat. I started to get a little bitter, and that was something I'd promised I'd never get, so it was time to seek out a new horizon.

My self-esteem had dipped so low that it was almost impossible to decide on what to do. It couldn't involve too much contact with the public because people might recognise me and I didn't have the energy to answer the barrage of questions: 'What are you doing here?', 'Couldn't you get another job?', 'How much did you get paid in *Hollyoaks*?'

But I wasn't much of a typist either, and by this point I felt I was too unsightly for anybody to want me on their reception. I was in a serious rut.

A friend of mine, Joan, was over from Belfast and she insisted I accompany her to a wedding reception of somebody I'd never met. I really wasn't in the mood for a wedding but wanted to see Joan while she was over.

At the wedding, the bride marched over and in a thick

Belfast accent asked, 'Did you used to be in *Hollyoaks*?' Before I could confirm or deny, she continued, 'You left ages ago. What are you doing now?' This question was starting to sting more and more each time I was asked.

'Er . . . nothing. I'm trying to decide what I fancy doing,' I muttered.

On the spot she offered me a job, and there started my career as a recruitment consultant.

The very same day I received my contract of employment in the post, I also received a letter from my agent. This was the first time she had contacted me in four months.

> It is with great regret that I have to send this letter, but I have been asked to streamline my list. Unfortunately, with the current climate being as it is, I find myself in a difficult situation.
>
> I know this will come as a shock, and of course please feel free to call me. It goes without saying that we'll still handle any enquiries that come in for you until you find new representation.
>
> Wishing you all the best . . .

So that is how one is fired by one's agent. I had to laugh at her use of words. She found herself in a 'difficult situation'! I'd say that mine was far more problematic.

It was summer 2005, I'd had a year of unemployment and now had no agent. I wondered if I'd ever act again, but I refused to give up hope. I had no choice but to take a non-acting job to pay my mortgage. I knew my time would come again and that something would show up when I least expected it to. I was right.

22

A Disingenuous Gastric Band

19 stone 6 pounds

By autumn 2005 I was quite settled in my new job and resigned to remaining there until Spielberg or Scorsese came knocking. And then I got a call.

To be more precise, it was a message on my mobile to call Carolyn at Granada. Naturally intrigued, I returned her call immediately. She chatted away to me about mundane things.

After five minutes I began to wonder why she had contacted me. I decided it was time to be assertive. 'So, how can I help?' I asked.

There was a pregnant pause, then she said, 'Er, well, we were wondering if you would like to, or be interested in, or consider . . . Now don't bite my head off . . .*Celebrity Fit Club.*'

I suppose this isn't the easiest of calls to make, as some people are in complete denial about their appearance. I could have flipped out or replied stroppily, 'Are you saying I'm fat?' But instead I simply said, 'Yes.'

She was over the moon. I think she was slightly taken aback because she had a well-rehearsed pitch about having access to the best nutritionist in the country and the best fitness advice, and thought she'd have to work very hard to persuade me. Instead she found me fired up with enthusiasm at the very mention of the words '*Celebrity Fit Club*'.

'That's fabulous, really fabulous,' she said. 'Let's fix a date to have lunch with my producer and talk the whole thing through.'

I was very excited at the prospect of appearing on *Celebrity Fit Club*. As well as an opportunity to raise my public profile, I welcomed the chance to embark on an exercise and fitness programme that I knew had been life-changing for others. As with the documentary that never was, I knew that I responded well to public challenges of this kind. I was confident that I could rise to the occasion. I was looking forward to getting started already. I wasn't happy with the way my eating habits were deteriorating and the pointer on my scales was creeping up. I knew I needed to take action. The call couldn't have come at a better time for me.

I had previously been asked to go on Dr Gillian McKeith's *You Are What You Eat* but had said no because I was worried that she might humiliate me. I'm not keen on her patronising approach. I recently met Gillian on *Big Brother's Little Brother*, and even at 16 stone I like to think I look healthier than she does – I guess I'm biased, though.

Carolyn and I duly set a date to meet. I rarely took a lunchbreak at work, but obviously this was one occasion where a lunchbreak was in order.

My boss at the recruitment consultancy had recently criticised my performance at work. 'You're not very motivated,' he had said. 'You need to start thinking about the money more. Every phone call you make is going to make you more money. You need to start thinking about your back pocket.' I knew that I should take his comments on board.

Carolyn had selected an Italian restaurant. As we walked in, food and weight thoughts jabbered through my brain: Oh, my God, what should I order? Should I impress them that I've already turned over a new nutritional leaf and order a *salade niçoise*? Or should I choose something unhealthy and fattening so they'll think I'll be a real challenge? And what about when they bring a basket of bread? Should I take some, or refuse it? Should I put butter on it, or ask for olive oil to show how aware I am of healthy eating?

And so my monologue went on. It was deafening me by the time I arrived at the table and shook hands with Carolyn and her producer, Tim.

We all got along very well. I ate heartily, stopped worrying about what they thought of me, and we laughed about diets and brutal exercise regimes. I became very excited about the prospect of being on *Celebrity Fit Club*. I knew from the successful diet I'd gone on when the sumo film fell through and the hard work I'd put into the fitness and weight-loss documentary that never was with Dave that I'd be able to rise to the challenge.

I'd told my colleagues in the office that I'd be back in an hour, but the lunch extended to two and a quarter hours.

'Where have you been?' my boss demanded, when I got back to the office.

For once I had the perfect answer: 'I've been thinking more about my back pocket.' I smirked. He had no answer to that.

Unfortunately I didn't think enough about income-generating opportunities from *Celebrity Fit Club*. I didn't have an agent at that time. Carolyn had explained that the participants were paid according to their level of celebrity and that I ranked somewhere in the middle. She wouldn't tell me who else was being considered and said that negotiations were still ongoing. She also said, 'We've got a back-up for every demographic except yours.'

At that point those money thoughts that my boss was encouraging me to have should have kicked in, but alas they didn't. They'd asked me first and they didn't have a back-up with a similar profile to mine – I should have bargained for more than what they said they'd pay me. We all had to have a medical check-up before embarking on our weight-loss quest. Dr Adam Carey, the show's doctor and nutritionist, had rooms in Harley Street.

He was a pleasant, professional man and took careful notes of my medical history, including what I ate and drank and whether I smoked. I was appalled when I calculated that I drank more than a hundred units of alcohol a week, but was congratulated for having given up smoking.

He asked me about the medical history of my siblings.

'Well, one sister died of bowel cancer, the other one is slightly mental, but my brother's OK,' I said.

He allowed himself a small smile.

I told him that I suffered from agonisingly painful periods that had got gradually worse over the years to the point where the pain caused me to throw up and pass out. He suggested that losing weight would probably help.

'The reason that lots of overweight women suffer badly with certain aspects of their periods is related to their body-fat percentage. Women naturally have more body fat than men because this is one of the deciding factors in the amount of oestrogen produced. Therefore excess body fat can cause your body to overproduce oestrogen, creating a hormone imbalance that will in turn affect your periods,' he said.

This new information fascinated me. Had I known this sooner, it would surely have given me much-needed motivation to lose weight. As it turns out, I actually have endometriosis, which I am currently being treated for, so hopefully by the time you read this, the days of my horrendous period pains will be long gone.

'What's your ideal weight?' he asked me.

'I suppose around fifteen stone,' I said. 'All I want to be able to do is to go to any shop on the high street and buy size-sixteen clothes.'

He raised his eyebrows, apparently disappointed that I was aiming so low in terms of my weight loss.

'In terms of my acting work, I don't want to become too slim. I've established myself as an overweight actress, and people are going to come looking for me for that. I'm always going to be a character actress because I'm six foot tall, so why not be fat and tall. And then there's the ginger taboo. Don't tell me you want me to dye my hair blonde just so I look like everybody else!' I said. 'And don't forget if I lose too much weight, I'll have yards and yards of excess skin to lug around with me.'

Poor Adam hadn't managed to get a word in. I hoped I'd presented an open-and-shut case for why I didn't want to lose too much weight.

On my way to the first *Celebrity Fit Club* meeting on 11 December 2005, I decided to treat myself to a last supper at a McDonald's drive-thru. Throwing caution to the wind, I ordered a double quarter-pounder with cheese, large fries, a chocolate doughnut, a McFlurry ice cream and six chicken nuggets with sweet curry sauce. I had a hangover and it's at times like that that McDonald's food tastes particularly good. Since doing *Celebrity Fit Club* I've only succumbed to the temptation of McDonald's once and didn't even finish it.

The venue for our fitness training was Bisham Abbey, not far from Reading. It's a beautiful location and looks particularly stunning on bleak winter days.

Everyone else had already arrived by the time I got there and had changed into their gym clothes. I soon discovered that we weren't actually going to get weighed until the beginning of January – the traditional time for New Year's resolutions to kick in.

I couldn't wait to see who the other contestants were. I already knew 'Quinny' (Micky Quinn). But I was very nervous when I saw a crowd of new faces – some I recognised and some I didn't. One of the contestants was Sharon Marshall. She had a shock of hair dyed a fluorescent shade of claret. Anne Diamond, Russell Grant, Carole Malone, Jeff Rudom and Bobby George were the others.

I was expecting pep talks, diet sheets and an introduction to punishing workouts. Instead, everything was very low key, a sort of anticlimax before we'd even begun. After we'd lined up together, we were ushered out into a lush, green field. Russell Grant had hurt his foot. He looked very unwell and was limping badly. Apparently he was recovering from a chest infection too.

I knew Quinny because he's a regular at Jalon's and an old friend of the owner. I knew he would be great fun and that he would be the one to keep all our spirits high. Like everyone else, I felt I knew Anne Diamond a tiny bit from

TV AM and because of the very public bereavement she suffered when she lost one of her sons to cot death. It's a very strange feeling knowing about someone's sad loss when you don't know them personally. I didn't know whether I should say an extremely belated, 'I'm very sorry for your loss,' or not acknowledge what had happened in any way. In the end I decided to keep my mouth shut.

Jeff Rudom was a man I hadn't come across before. He was American and weighed a whopping 32 stone 7 pounds. On first sight he didn't appeal to me, but I forced myself to try and put my reservations on hold and not make a snap judgement about him.

We were ushered out on to the freezing-cold field. Harvey, our fitness trainer, looked gleeful.

'Right, what fatties have I got today?' he said. As if he didn't know.

I was irritated by his remark and vowed that I was going to prove myself by working incredibly hard at exercising and losing weight.

He picked a fight with Russell immediately. 'What are you doing with that stick?' he barked.

'I need the stick because I can't walk,' said Russell, wondering why he was having to state the blindingly obvious. 'And by the way, the trainers in my room are the wrong size.'

My heart sank. Russell was a lovely, cuddly memory from my childhood. I hoped the reality of him wouldn't prove to be a terrible disappointment. Harvey instructed us to jog round the field, which we did at varying speeds and with varying degrees of wobble from our surplus flesh. The run was only a gentle one, a warm-up I think Harvey called it, but quite a few people panted and sweated over it.

Then we were led back inside. I was mystified when we were taken into a room that contained a table groaning with fattening, unhealthy food – pizza, pork pies, chicken drumsticks and mayonnaise-laden sandwiches. I looked up and surprise, surprise, there were cameras capturing our movements from every angle.

Time for the gratuitous shots of fat people feeding their faces, I thought to myself grimly. I felt defiant and was the first one to get myself a plate of food. In gatherings of 'normal-sized' people, I never wanted to be the first one to bolt for the buffet, but I decided that because some of the people in this particular gathering were bigger than me, it really didn't matter.

I thought that if I lost a stone before the show started properly in January, I'd have a head start. Over Christmas, however, my good intentions fell by the wayside and instead of losing a stone I put on another stone. The doctor, Adam, had actually cautioned me against losing weight before the show started because then I would plateau at the beginning of filming and he had feared I might get disheartened if my weight loss was at a slower pace than everyone else's. Just as well, then, I suppose, that I gained a stone rather than lost it.

In January, we were invited to participate in team-building exercises. It was still very unclear exactly how things were going to work. We stayed in a beautiful hotel near the abbey each Saturday night that the show was filmed. We arrived there at Saturday lunchtime and spent around twenty-four hours there. For the rest of the week it was up to us to motivate ourselves in the course of our daily lives and to get on with whichever exercise programme we had decided to pursue. I continued working in the recruitment consultancy while I did *Celebrity Fit Club*.

Anne and Carole were appointed team captains. I hadn't realised it but they had carved up the teams beforehand, and although it was supposed to look spontaneous, both knew exactly who was on their team. Carole chose Sharon, and Anne chose me. Then Carole picked Bobby, and Anne picked Russell, so Quinny and Jeff were left.

'Pick Quinny, Anne,' I urged.

'We'll see,' she said.

It had already been decided that we would have Jeff, but of course I didn't know this. The pretence of picking out team members was purely a manufactured exercise for the benefit of the cameras.

Amy Lamé came on the show to interview all of us about our weight-loss aspirations. 'So, Mikyla, how much weight would you like to lose?'

'I'd like to get down to around fifteen stone, maybe fourteen. I'm aiming to be a size sixteen,' I said.

Harvey, the fitness instructor, looked at me scornfully. 'You know what, Mikyla, I don't know if you're going to make it because I don't think you want it enough.'

Whilst it no doubt made good TV, this infuriated me. Just because I wasn't rushing at him begging him to turn me into a Barbie doll, it somehow translated into me being unlikely to succeed. The fact that I wasn't clutching a picture of myself as a size-10 sylph wearing a swimsuit somehow made me a less worthwhile candidate. I know I'm in the minority and most fat people would donate their internal organs if they were offered a slim body, but not me. I've been fat throughout my life and of course it has caused me some distress but I've still had an amazing time, one that some could only dream of, so why should I be preoccupied with being 'normal' or 'average'?

I wanted to scream, 'Piss off.' Instead I stared right at him and said, 'Well, we'll see about that.'

Anne was supportive: 'You'll do well, Mikyla, because for you this is about clothes and shopping and that will motivate you.'

'Yes, it will,' I said. 'All I want is to be a size sixteen.'

As soon as the cameras stopped rolling, Dr Adam asked for a 'word'. We walked into a smaller room, where a different camera was waiting for us. He sat me down like a head teacher and lectured me about not having had my pre-show blood test. I genuinely hadn't had a chance to do it.

'My holiday from work runs from January to January and I'd used up every single day. Now it's January again, I could book a day off and have the blood test done,' I explained, apologising for not having done it back in December. 'My failure to have a blood test is not an indication that I don't want to make major changes. I'm really cross that Harvey's suggesting I'm lazy because I don't want to be an size ten.'

'He never said that.'

'He implied it.'

'Well, go away and lose weight and prove us wrong,' he said.

'I genuinely want to lose weight. I just need to know what the rules are,' I said.

'First go up to Harley Street and get your blood test done and then we'll see about the rules.'

When I got the results of my blood test, I couldn't believe

how healthy I was considering my weight. My cholesterol levels were slightly high but certainly not off the scale, and to everyone's surprise, including mine, my liver was in fine fettle despite the enormous amount of alcohol that I regularly consumed – Dr Adam said he was 'relieved but shocked' at its good condition. I was also given the all-clear for diabetes.

We were then all taken to the canteen for a talk about healthy eating. Most of us knew what the basics of healthy eating were but just didn't bother to abide by them.

'What you need to be able to identify are fibrous carbs, starchy carbs and protein,' said Dr Adam. 'You need to eat equal weights of all three.'

There was only one meal that I was able to cook from scratch – stir-fried chicken with onions and peppers. In fact I ate this meal more or less every day for four months.

We were urged to replace evil processed white bread, rice and pasta with the healthy wholegrain varieties.

To me, this way of eating was absolutely revolutionary. It was different from any of the diets I had been on before. On day one, fired up with good intentions, I marched off purposefully to Tesco in Canary Wharf and resolved to fill my basket with the kinds of foods Dr Adam would approve of. But it was easier said than done. Everything I picked up seemed to be too salty, too sugary, too processed, or if it was fresh and raw, beyond my limited culinary capabilities to turn it into something edible.

'This is going to be horrendous,' I said to myself. 'I'll end up eating absolutely nothing – I'll be the first *Celebrity Fit Club* contestant to starve to death!' I walked around for twenty minutes placing things in my basket only to have to remove them seconds later as another one of Dr Adam's restrictions leapt into my mind. I seriously thought my head was going to explode. Just imagine how many calories that would burn! By this point I was ridiculously hungry. I was going through sugar and caffeine cold turkey and was totally exasperated at the lack of anything suitable for lunch.

The result was a 6-foot, 19-stone redhead bursting into floods of tears. Part of me wanted to lie on the floor kicking and screaming like a two-year-old having a tantrum. I reminded myself that if it was easy to lose weight, we wouldn't have such a growing obesity epidemic in this country.

When I'd left the supermarket, I decided to ring fellow contestant Sharon to see if she was struggling as much as I was.

'There's nothing I can eat,' I barked down the phone.

She sounded calm and composed. 'Didn't you read the sheet?' she said.

'No, what sheet?'

This is where I take after my mother. Her approach is 'Who needs to read instructions? They're such a waste of time. Just forge ahead and you'll figure it out.'

Er, no, I don't think so – not this time.

'Sorry, Sharon, can you tell me what's on it, then maybe I can go back to the supermarket and buy some sodding food?'

She ran through what I could and couldn't have. I brightened at the prospect of being able to eat half a baked potato for lunch.

We all had to join a gym as part of our fitness regime. I managed to blag six months' free membership at Holmes Place, Canary Wharf. It was lovely – far nicer than my own home – with its heated floors and Molton Brown cosmetics in the changing rooms. This made it much more inviting at stupid o'clock in the morning.

One of the most valuable things that Harvey instructed us to do for the duration of *Celebrity Fit Club* and then for the rest of our lives was to go into 'mental lockdown' so that our minds moved to a different place – a land where vigorous exercise was a way of life most days, where sugar and refined carbohydrates were banished to some hinterland never to be visited again. Porridge with honey for breakfast was the highlight of my day and it was substantial enough to see me through till lunch, because oats are carbs that release energy slowly.

Three days into the fitness regime, not only did my stomach think my throat had been cut, but I had a splitting headache that had kicked in on the first day. I couldn't understand why I felt so bad.

One of the guys at work, Matt, could see that I was about to climb up the office wall because I was being deprived of everything: no sugar, no fat, no Diet Coke, no alcohol, no tea.

'Wait a minute – tea?' I'm sure you're thinking. In truth, there is nothing whatsoever wrong with tea, but it wasn't listed on the information sheet, so I figured that just like all my other addictions it was contraband. I sat there looking longingly at my colleague's perfectly-brewed cup of tea.

'Give me that doctor's number,' Matt said. 'I need to have a word with him about this tea malarkey. I can't handle four months of this – it's worse than PMT. You can't deprive people of a cup of tea.'

In the end I decided to email Dr Adam.

He responded swiftly by phone. 'Who gave you the impression you couldn't have tea?'

As I tried to explain myself on the phone, I could hear my colleague Matt mumbling at the kettle to hurry up and boil in order to get some much-needed caffeine inside me. I think this was a turning point between myself and the doc. It was the point when he realised I was deadly serious about my determination to shed the equivalent of a sack of potatoes.

'Poor you,' he said. 'If you've cut out all caffeine and all fats and sugars, you must be in a living hell right now.'

'It's so bad I can't even discuss it – I'll call you back after my cuppa!' I said.

As I put the phone down, Matt handed me the best cup of tea I'd ever tasted. Instantly my pounding headache eased. It was quite scary how the caffeine fix from the tea soothed my withdrawal symptoms. I had become addicted to caffeine without having the slightest idea.

When we arrived at the abbey on Saturday afternoon at the end of our first week, we had our weekly weigh-in. I hadn't been on the scales all week but was expecting them to show a spectacular weight loss because I had been 100 per cent virtuous on the diet and exercise front. I remember in the car journey there Sharon was swilling water around her mouth to relieve her thirst but spitting it out instead of swallowing it to ensure she didn't add extra ounces. We actually got weighed before filming began, as the most accurate scales are not quite in keeping with the décor of the abbey and need to be calibrated. That said, we did not see the reading, so when we mounted the giant fake scales on set, they were in our minds the true scales. They left me until last. I started to panic a little. I knew there had to be some drama or other to it. Adam and Harvey both looked very grave. I was growing increasingly concerned that maybe, despite making a superhuman effort, I'd lost no weight. Feelings of prickly horror crept down my spine.

Surely I've lost something, I thought. Something . . .

Then the suspense was over. I'd only gone and lost 10 bloody pounds. I was astounded. I didn't believe that kind of weight loss was possible in a week. I was so elated and overwhelmed, I didn't even have the inclination to gloat to Harvey, 'I told you so.' All my trauma had been worth it. I was over the moon and incredibly motivated to succeed.

I continued religiously with my routine of early-morning sessions at the gym, and although it was the purest form of tastebud torture known to mankind, instead of making a beeline for the doughnut stand close to my office, I walked past it, trying not to even inhale the delicious fumes of fried sweet batter that wafted towards my nostrils. I didn't allow myself to look those doughnuts in the eye and instead headed purposefully towards the miso-soup stand. To my amazement, my tastebuds started to adapt and my zero tolerance towards chocolate, alcohol and fatty foods paid off.

Various frictions were developing between certain individuals in the show. Carole accused Anne of making lots of money out of her dieting trials and tribulations, though Anne would have argued this was the last thing she was doing. Jeff was increasingly disliked by almost everyone. Russell became more and more lovable as the show progressed. At the beginning of the show he felt unwell, and perhaps this made him feel more vulnerable than usual. But he is a warm-hearted, lovely man, and he really got stuck in with everybody else. Anne seemed very reluctant to take part in many of the physical challenges, and we didn't find out why until later. Increasingly she was distancing herself from the rest of us. The other contestants were critical of her, but I had inherited the quality from my dad of championing the underdog, and simply because so many of the others were grumbling about her, I felt disinclined to join in.

Instead I sat on the fence where opinions about Anne were concerned – a very unusual position for me to adopt, I can tell you. Usually no one can stop me expressing strong and vocal views about everything under the sun.

One of the toughest tests assigned to us was when Harvey took a week off and two replacement army fitness instructors were drafted in to take his place. My competitive streak kicked in. The two teams were made to run in relays holding extremely heavy medicine balls. Various team members dropped out and only Bobby, Sharon, Quinny and I were left. We had to crawl through stinking undergrowth. We were absolutely filthy by the end of it, and I felt more physically exhausted than I could ever remember feeling before.

When he got back from his week off, Harvey became very exasperated with Anne when he learned how she'd refused to take part in the army-style assault course. 'A team captain needs to lead from the front,' he said to her. 'You're fired.'

Anne seemed prepared for this. She looked very upset but was very professional.

Then talk turned to a replacement for Anne. Almost everyone said that I should step into the role, including Anne. 'Mikyla should be my replacement,' she said. 'She has worked so hard and she's an inspiration to everyone.'

'It's got to be Miky,' Russell chimed in. 'She's young and she's vibrant.'

Then Jeff spoke up in his ridiculously slow drawl. I wondered if he had got so big because it was easier for him to eat than speak.

'I suppose it should be Mikyla because she's more popular than me, although I do think that I would do a good job,' he said.

Then the presenter, Dale Winton, asked me who I thought should be team captain.

'Well, that's a very difficult one for me to answer,' I said. 'I think it should be someone who leads by example.'

I assumed that I would be made the new captain, but in the interests of creating friction on the show and, they hoped, better TV, they decided against putting me into the hot seat.

'Mikyla, you have really impressed us. Jeff, you don't have the right attitude at the moment, but we've decided to make you the new team captain.'

I sat there gasping, clutching my obligatory 'time of the month' hot-water bottle. 'That's absolutely ridiculous,' I said. 'Anne had the captaincy taken away from her because she didn't complete the physical challenges you set us. But Jeff didn't complete them either.'

I was enraged not because I hadn't been chosen but because of the hypocrisy of the whole thing.

Then Jeff made one of his slow, infuriating pronouncements. 'I know what you're saying is right, Mikyla, so I'm going to have you as my deputy captain.'

'Don't be ridiculous,' I said. 'You're the captain – you need to get on with this.' Then I walked out of the room.

Afterwards I wanted to kick myself for rising to the bait the show's producers had set, but that's the curse of being ginger. Containing a temper tantrum isn't always possible.

Later I took Harvey aside and in front of the cameras said, 'What really annoys me about all of this is that you set yourself up as someone who cared about us but we have all rolled over for the "product".'

Harvey looked at me impassively.

'I didn't want to be team captain and I don't care about any of that, but I think that you have undermined your credibility.'

At that point the cameras stopped rolling. They weren't interested in filming any criticism of the fundamental way the show worked. I carried on.

Jeff turned out to be as bad as the rest of us had feared. He insisted at shouting at us in a monotone, 'C'mon, c'mon, c'mon,' and calling us to talk about himself for hours on end. We started to avoid his calls.

Anne and I took him aside to address the shouting issue. The two of us got along well, and she was very warm and motherly towards me.

'Look, Jeff,' we said to him, 'you've got to stop shouting. It really doesn't work for us.' He shrugged and didn't take what we said on board.

The following Saturday we were all instructed that the cameras would be joining us for breakfast in the hotel at 7 a.m. the next morning. We speculated about why this was but had no clue. Anne had opted to stay at home on the Saturday night as she was within commuting distance, so it was the remaining seven of us who had been asked to attend. Then the producers came in, looking grave. When we saw

Tim, the executive producer, we knew it must be something serious for him to be out of his bed at this hour on a Sunday.

'We've got a very serious announcement to make about Anne,' Tim said.

My heart skipped a beat. I thought that something terrible had happened to her. Maybe she'd collapsed or something.

'She's had surgery,' he continued.

Again I panicked for her. Maybe she'd had an emergency appendix removal, perforated ulcer—

'She had a gastric band fitted.'

'When did she have that done?' I asked in an unusually bimbo-like manner.

'What's that got to do with the price of mincemeat?' said Quinny, rolling his eyes.

Carole sat there working out what her reaction should be. Then she spoke. 'I'm sorry, but that's bloody out-rageous. It's cheating!'

'That's not right. This is a competition and she's given herself an unfair advantage,' said Sharon.

'She's a cheating bastard,' said Bobby bluntly. Quinny and Bobby were united on this one. As sportsmen, they viewed unfair advantages over opponents very seriously. After a moment's consideration, Bobby added, 'She should have had a tit job instead – at least she could have seen what she got for her money.' That comment did raise a chuckle – trust Bobby to say something like that. We now also understood why Anne had held back from some of the physical challenges – because of the operation, she couldn't take part.

I did understand where everyone was coming from, but somehow didn't have the heart to agree with them. I felt that unanimous condemnation was a little too harsh to dish out to somebody who clearly had 'issues'.

'Don't you feel sorry for her?' I asked. Everybody looked at me as if I was mad. 'Secretly getting a gastric band fitted is a really sad thing to do,' I continued.

Carole was quick to contradict me. 'Don't kid yourself, Mikyla. She knew exactly what she was doing.' Then she flicked on the journalist switch. It was like the floodlights at Old Trafford suddenly being snapped on. She started to fire questions at Tim: 'When did she tell you? Why did she tell you? Which tabloids know?' She was already reaching for her mobile to call the *Mirror* news desk.

Even though I'd known from the outset that Sharon and Carole were tabloid journalists, it wasn't until that moment I linked up the fact that people doing a job that I had always thought was only for the lowest of the low were my friends, who happened to be warm, kind human beings, rather than having the cold, vicious qualities that I had assumed were part of the job description.

'At the end of the day, what Anne has done highlights the fact that her problem is far more serious than any of ours,' I said. 'I want to lose weight as much as everyone else, but I know that if I don't lose another pound until the day I die, I'll still be happy.'

'Don't be soft,' said Quinny. 'People are going to think she's a cheat and you're going to come off looking stupid cos you can't see it.'

'I believe what you're saying is right,' I said. 'But I don't like this feeling that there's a lynch mob out to get Anne.'

There was all sorts of talk about Anne's gastric band, that it hadn't been fitted right and that's why she wasn't losing weight, or that she was swallowing liquidised Mars bars and ice cream. The producers had told us about the gastric band because the *News of the World* was about to break the story. Anne had gone to a Belgian clinic to have the band fitted, and another UK woman who was having one fitted at the same time had spotted Anne and got on the phone to the *News of the World.*

We all sat around a table and waited for Anne to arrive. My stomach was churning for her at the thought of how nervous she must be, having to face all of us.

We greeted her in a civilised way. Nobody grabbed her by the throat or hurled insults at her. We just quizzed her about her reasons and asked her to explain why she'd done what she did. Carole took the lead and then we all followed her calm, direct style of questioning.

We were asked if we wanted Anne to stay or go. Although the general feeling was disapproval, nobody wanted her to leave. I even cried as she talked of writing letters to her sons before going under the anaesthetic. But by the same token nobody felt like begging her to stay.

Anne felt terribly humiliated and walked out distraught after she'd made her statement to us all. In the end she chose to leave the show. I suppose it was inevitable, and it certainly made for dramatic telly.

I sent her a text saying, 'Please don't do anything rash. You've got to come back and show them you're a fighter.'

Her response was, 'You've got to be one of the kindest people. Thank you for your support and friendship.'

Strangely, despite several attempts to contact her, I never heard from Ms Diamond again. Oh, well, it's never too late . . . My number hasn't changed, Anne!

As the show went on, other people had started to notice how much weight I was losing. I think there's a real etiquette to commenting on weight loss. I much preferred it when people said things like, 'You look really well – you've lost weight,' rather than, 'You look so much better than you did before', as that means you looked awful before and makes you defensive. I've always been big; I've never been small and slender and I know I never will be. I've managed to accept that about myself, so why can't others?

Thanks to embarking on *Celebrity Fit Club*, I was gaining an insight into the mechanics of exercise and the importance of eating precisely. A few years ago I could gain a stone and nobody would really notice, but now that I'd lost weight, any weight gain would be more obvious.

As the weeks on the show passed, we all became much closer. There was a lot of laughter and banter. In the week that my period was due, I lost no weight at all. I was gutted.

Dr Adam said, 'Don't worry, that's perfectly normal, it's all down to water retention. Do you want to talk about it on the show? If you don't, the viewers might think that you've been cheating. It'll be comforting to other women who are dieting and are in the same situation as you.'

I wasn't particularly keen to have it announced on the telly that I hadn't lost any weight because my period was due, but I knew that it would ruin my morale, not to mention brand me as a diet cheat, not to tell the truth.

OK, I said to myself, taking a deep breath, I'm the ambassador for periods this week!

I even walked past a building site on the way in to work the day after the show had aired to a chorus of 'All right, darlin'? Got the decorators in, 'av we?' Great. Just what I needed at seven thirty in the morning.

I lost a bit more weight after my period week, but then, although I continued with the programme, the weight loss stopped again.

I got on the phone to Dr Adam about the fat that simply wouldn't budge.

He tried to calm me down. 'There are times when your body has had enough of losing weight,' he said. 'You're trying to turn a tank into a BMW and there's going to be some resistance. One thing you can do is remove the starchy carbs just for a few weeks and abandon your morning bowl of porridge.'

I was gutted. The porridge was the only meal I really enjoyed at that point. 'What am I going to eat instead?' I said, horrified.

'Well, you could make yourself something protein-based like an omelette,' he said. Grudgingly I agreed to abandon my filling porridge for a while and to try making myself omelettes.

My routine was to go to the gym before work and then make myself some breakfast in the office kitchen. As I've mentioned before, however, cooking isn't my forté. I managed to spectacularly burn the omelette and set off the fire alarm at work. We were all evacuated and had to stand outside in the freezing cold. Needless to say, my colleagues weren't best pleased with me. To add insult to injury, there was a callout fee of several hundred pounds that had to be paid to the fire brigade because it was a false alarm. The sum was deducted from our commission.

In my quest to shift more stubborn pounds of flesh, I had taken to working out at both the beginning and the end of the day.

To my delight, by the end of the four months, I had gone from morbidly obese to clinically obese to just obese. Sharon had gone from obese to her ideal weight, and Quinny went from morbidly obese to just overweight and was declared the programme's winner.

Five of us went out for a meal to celebrate at the end of the show. There was wonderful food on offer, and after our diet rations it all tasted so good. We managed to get through nine bottles of champagne and five bottles of wine between us. I personally polished off two bottles of champagne, a bottle of wine and substantial quantities of vodka.

My hangover the next morning was off the scale. I was shaking, I felt sick, and the inside of my mouth felt like a pair of trainers.

Once my hangover wore off, I was able to appreciate just how wonderful and life-changing an experience going on *Celebrity Fit Club* had been. I had been wary of losing too much weight, firstly because I would be plagued with too many folds of loose, redundant skin hanging off my body, and secondly because if I got my weight really low, I would no longer be able to hide it if I gained a few extra pounds. I enjoyed the comfort of my body hiding a few pounds here or there without people noticing.

What really mattered, though, was that as a result of *Celebrity Fit Club*, even though I hadn't won the race, at long last I was in it. For the first time in years I weighed 16 stone.

Epilogue

Writing this book has been an extraordinary experience that has forced me to undergo a form of DIY therapy. I have really had to look deep inside myself in order to understand why my relationship with food presents a daily struggle that I constantly need to overcome.

I guess some of it is down to greed, some of it comes from being self-destructive and some of it is down to my strange relationship with my dad. Thankfully I can control my greed and have grown out of the self-destruct phase. My relationship with my dad is still up and down but far more stable than it used to be. I know he loves me but by his own admission doesn't understand the concept of unconditional love. Maybe that's what I've been longing for all this time and I need to accept a person can't give what they don't have. My mum is the opposite and has lavished me with love and affection. As a result she is my absolute best friend and without her I couldn't have dealt with what life has thrown at me. She has instilled a real sense of self-belief in me and given me the confidence to barge into a skinny world and make it 'OK' to be fat.

As it stands my commitment to exercise is consistent although the motivational side often needs tweaking, so I have to invent new ways to keep my exercise regime interesting. On a recent trip to France Jay and I did an equipment inventory before we set off, that included boxing gloves, boxing pads, two skipping ropes and a medicine ball. Despite consuming copious amounts of wine and cheese we did manage to train every morning with my nephews George and Henry cheering us on and chanting the theme from *Rocky*. We had to laugh at how much things have changed from the days of running round the park in Blackburn with Jay screaming at me to get a move on. I'm now the one wanting to do an extra ten minuites. I can only hope that I hold on to my resolve, as I am positive that exercise is the key to weight maintenance. It allows me the odd blow out without gaining those dreaded few pounds that always seem to appear around my midriff, which for me symbolises the step from curvy to fat.

My relationship with food is still turbulent but knowledge is power, so thanks to Dr Adam I am much better equipped to regain control when I hit free-fall. I still enjoy food immensely and can be regularly distracted by thoughts of it and how good it will taste. To combat this I try to prepare meals in advance, that way I don't ponder what I fancy for dinner from 3 o'clock in the afternoon and I'm not tempted to falter because I already know what dinner is. We could all conquer our weight problem if we had a 24-hour chef and a hunky fitness instructor waiting to train us at 6 am every morning but the reality is we don't. Still, we can beat this monster down single-handed if we really want it enough.

Now, I'm not talking about becoming the far too-publicised size zero! Who wants to be malnourished and de-sexed? I'm talking about being happy and healthy. I am not suggesting people can't be both fat and happy because heaven knows I was during certain periods of my life, but being obese or worse still, morbidly obese does nobody any favours. It shortens your life expectancy and makes your day-to-day existence more problematic. If you're avoiding staircases like the plague and having to ask for seatbelt extensions on flights, then something needs to be done.

I was inspired by Jamie Oliver's recent endeavour to sort out the nation's school dinners as it is a fundamental issue and can definitely help combat the growing epidemic of childhood obesity. It is vital that we raise awareness of how important a healthy nutritious balanced diet is, and that we don't allow our taste buds to become addicted to sweet-tasting food. So many parents are unwittingly feeding their children refined carbohydrates and hydrodgenated fats – it's as if these kids exist in a sea of processed food. I really hope that the days of the fast-food giants are numbered but I fear they are here to stay.

Successfully losing weight and keeping it off has been a life-altering experience. I feel like so many doors have opened for me – particularly the all important retail doors, as shopping for clothes is now so much easier. Suranne and I used to dream about starting a clothing line aimed at big-busted, curvaceous women. We used to sketch designs and I think on one occasion after a few glasses of vino, we even drew up a business plan. Maybe after this book that can be my next venture – watch this space?

Unfortunately, losing weight hasn't opened the door to Speilberg's office but we can live in hope that casting directors will become braver and strive to project a more realistic image of today's female population. My latest quest is to somehow get my voluptuous frame on the dance floor of *Strictly Come Dancing* and shake my ample booty!

I currently weigh 15st 3lbs and have set myself one last target. I want to reach 14st for my thirtieth birthday later this year. Anything less than 14st is beyond my comprehension and I fear would be too hard to maintain. In all honesty, if I don't lose another pound till the day I die that's fine by me. I'm sure plenty of people still consider me fat but I couldn't really give two hoots – I have accepted who I am and don't feel the need to be slim.

I don't have a problem with naturally slim people even if they do insist on wandering around in a bikini – good for them! I do however have a big problem with the negative images society is fed, especially teenagers. I'm thinking of the endless pages of stick-thin women, a large proportion of whom, endure a life of constant deprivation and are obsessive about weight to the point where you could question their sanity. Then, to make it worse, the celebrities who dare to be themselves and have fat days just like the rest of us, are all too often condemned in the press, leaving impressionable young girls and sometimes boys in fear of being chastised as result of being overweight. Whatever happened to being normal?

It is possible to be curvy, desirable and successful. From my experience most ordinary men, and by ordinary men I don't include the ones who spend untold hours in the gym honing their physique, I mean Joe Average, actually find confidence sexy and are a sucker for a killer smile. Which means so many of the publications that are marketed on being full of half-naked skinny women, are actually designed to fuel men's fantasies rather than represent what they are actually looking for in a women. This is what I keep telling myself anyway and thus far it has served me well.

There is also the issue of air brushing to be considered, where celebrities are airbrushed to enhance their already good looks. This can be a necessary evil to cover imperfections on the photograph itself but instead is frequently used to enhance the actual subject. This is another negative image that is unrealistic and that adds yet more pressure to conform.

I recently did a naked photo shoot for a magazine. When the initial request came in I was ready to say no until my agent Jaine explained that it was anti-size zero. I had to weigh up the pros and cons. I had become much more at ease with my body and was comfortable to be naked with my partner, not worrying what he thought of my wobbly bits – but this was different: a room full of strangers capturing hard evidence of my shortcomings and then sharing their findings with millions of people. I was by this point adamant I couldn't do it but then I started to think about the lack of positive images of overweight people and how much this troubled me. I realised this was my chance to put my money where my mouth was and possibly encourage people to be themselves and realise that we don't need to conform to the media's idea of aesthetic perfection. I agreed to do it. I have to admit the shoot was very challenging; my heart was racing the whole time – but boy, am I glad I did it. This is something I could never have done up until now and it did empower me especially as there wasn't an airbrush in sight!

For the first time in my life I'm in control of my weight instead of my weight being in control of me and I'll tell you – that feels great!

Acknowledgements

I am blessed to have so many incredible people around me and such wonderful memories but it has proved impossible to put all of them into this book so please don't think this is a reflection of their importance. To my mum: there are no words to express my gratitude so I won't embarrass myself trying – I love you five hundred twenty-five thousand six hundred minutes! Dad: I know so much of me is part of you and that has played a huge part in getting me to where I am today. I love you and don't think our difference needs to separate us. Jay, you're a top brother, all is forgiven. London Marathon here we come . . . ! x Sam, life's too short – the people we've lost are with us every day and wish us happiness. To all my little angels who often disguise themselves as mischievous little devils: Henry, George, India, Ashley, Lauren and Ellie, you bring a smile to my face every time I think of you. Not forgetting Simon and Claire with their party of five. Thanks for adopting me you nutters. Cameron and Preshella: 'You are the sunshine of my life, that's why I'll always be around' – I love you more than chocolate.

Thanks to Hodder & Stoughton, especially Rowena, for taking a gamble on this book, I hope it pays off for both our sakes. Nicola, thanks for always remaining calm even when

I was in a tizzy and helping me through the process. Diane, thanks for listening, it can't have been easy. Thank you to Lime Pictures for all their help and allowing us to use this title. Jaine, my agent and friend, you believed in the idea of this book more than I did so thank you but now you need to read the bloody thing.

David Johnson, I'd be here all day trying to list the wonderful things I have learned from you – thank you from the bottom of my heart, you are a legend in your own lifetime. Jo Hallows, you saw something so many others didn't, you opened a huge door for me and welcomed me in – thank you for the best four-and-a-half years of my life. Dave, I go to the gym four times a week, thank you for showing me the way. Adam, I have a healthy relationship with food and have beaten my addiction – I can't tell you how much that means to me. Thanks to the Hill McGlynn gang for supporting me and giving me the opportunity to build another career.

Gemma, my adopted kid sister, you are the fittest bitch I know but stay away from those footballers. Nick Pickard and your amazing family, I miss you! Russell the 'Ginger Ninja', you're the best house mate a girl could ask for. Julie Buckfield, you have the purest spirit and by the way, 'Catherine Zeta Jones won the Oscar'. To Terri and Sean, the coolest couple I know – it's all about Boxing day! To the Ibex house possie for giving me a 'local' Cheers. CFC crew, I couldn't have coped without you and all the laughter we shared. Gary, you are the most generous man I know and the first number I dial when I need somebody, thanks for picking up?! Sonia, a lifelong friend, you really do know every aspect of me and still love me – wow! And Andre, you left a handprint on my heart xx

Picture Credits

Most of the photographs are from the author's own collection. Additional sources: © Kenneth Barker 3 (top); © Lime Pictures 7 (top); © Rex 8 (top); © John Wright/Amarang.com 8 (bottom)

Every reasonable effort has been made to contact the copyright holders, but if there are any errors or omissions, Hodder & Stoughton will be pleased to insert the appropriate acknowledgement in any subsequent printing of this publication.